AUDITORY PERCEPTUAL DISORDERS

AUDITORY PERCEPTUAL DISORDERS

Second Edition

By

DAVID F. BARR, Ph.D.

Audiologist and Vice-President
Audiological Consultant
Associates, Incorporated
Oviedo, Florida

With a Foreword by

T. Walter Carlin, Ph.D.

Director
Sir Alexander Ewing Hearing & Speech Clinic
Ithaca College
Ithaca, New York

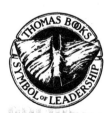

CHARLES C THOMAS • PUBLISHER
Springfield • *Illinois* • *U.S.A.*

Published and Distributed Throughout the World by
CHARLES C THOMAS • PUBLISHER
Bannerstone House
301-327 East Lawrence Avenue, Springfield, Illinois, U.S.A.

© *1976, by* CHARLES C THOMAS • PUBLISHER
ISBN 0-398-03411-7
Library of Congress Catalog Card Number: 76-6069

With THOMAS BOOKS *careful attention is given to all details of
manufacturing and design. It is the Publisher's desire to present books that are
satisfactory as to their physical qualities and artistic possibilities and
appropriate for their particular use.* THOMAS BOOKS *will be true to those
laws of quality that assure a good name and good will.*

Printed in the United States of America
R-1

Library of Congress Cataloging in Publication Data

Barr, David F
  Auditory perceptual disorders.

  Major portion of the 2d ed. is based on the
author's thesis, Patna University, India
  Bibliography: p.
  Includes index.
  1. Hearing disorders in children. 2. Auditory
perception. I. Title. [DNLM: 1. Auditory perception. 2. Perceptual disorders. WV272 B268a]
RF122.5.C4B37   1976   617.8′9   76-6069
ISBN 0-398-03411-7

This book is dedicated to my parents and to my teachers at the Baylor School, the University of Tennessee, and Patna University who stressed: AMAT VICTORIA CURAM

FOREWORD

IT is a rare privilege to have the opportunity to revise a Foreward to a text. Dr. Barr's book, *Auditory Perceptual Disorders,* has been developed in such a manner that it is sure to please the many different professionals working with children and adults. The straightforward style in which Dr. Barr approaches this difficult subject is refreshing. The inclusion of anatomy and physiology greatly strengthens the revised text.

Dr. Barr points out that assessment of auditory perceptual problems must too often await the onset of expressive difficulties in speech, reading, spelling and writing. He draws attention to auditory reception as a psycholinguistic function. He then presents a valuable step-by-step discussion of the nature and extent of auditory perceptual handicaps. This text should be most welcomed by busy physicians specializing in pediatrics, otology, neurology and psychiatry. Any worker who is involved with the well-being of the preschool child will find a great deal of experience and common sense has resulted in a most pragmatic approach to the problem.

The author's chapters on therapeutic considerations and classroom management come at a time when public school personnel are becoming increasingly aware of learning disabilities in the schools but have little training in how to identify and remediate the problem of auditory perceptual disorders. This book will appeal to the diagnostician, teacher and therapist.

This book should become part of the diagnostic and therapeutic battery of all workers involved with the hearing impaired. Particularly in the developing countries, the worker with the hearing impaired is one of the first to be approached when problems of auditory perception appear. This book will enable the professional and the layman to establish guidelines for an educational approach to auditory perceptual disorders in society.

Dr. Barr's text underlines and spotlights the prime importance of the auditory system in educating children in the ordinary school. I am pleased to recommend this text to all those throughout the world who work with children.

T. WALTER CARLIN

PREFACE

M Y purpose in writing this book has been to present an introduction to theories and practices in auditory perceptual disorders for a broad professional audience: special educators, speech and language pathologists, reading specialists, psychologists, optometrists, students and physicians as well as audiologists.

Many theoretical aspects of auditory perception are presented. Basic anatomy and physiology of the central nervous system, the physics of sound and the neuroendocrine control of perception are discussed. A glossary is provided to explain more exotic terminology. I have tried to avoid detailed remedial programs because good ones are readily available in other texts. Moreover, those who work with the perceptually handicapped child and who are well schooled in diagnostic and remedial procedures are, or should be, sufficiently imaginative and creative to set up a diagnostic-teaching program tailored to the specific needs of the individual child.

I have observed that far too little is known of receptive learning processes. I hope that the theories and practices discussed in this book will motivate professionals to undertake more, much needed research in the area of auditory perceptual disorders. I feel there has been a paucity of answers on this subject simply because few among the qualified have thought to ask the right questions. With these words of Lewis Carroll the author wishes the reader well on his quest for answers in auditory perception and its disorders:

> *"I said it very loud and clear*
> *I went and shouted in his ear*
> *And when I found the door was locked*
> *I pulled and pushed and kicked and knocked ...*

Auditory Perceptual Disorders

"It takes all the running you can do,
To keep in the same place.
If you want to get somewhere else,
You must run twice as fast as that!"

DAVID F. BARR

ACKNOWLEDGMENTS

I WISH to express my gratitude to the teachers, colleagues and friends who have contributed to the realization of this effort: Dr. David M. Lipscomb and Dr. Harold L. Luper, my professors at the University of Tennessee; Norman R. Carmel, M.A., Gloria Hall Nicholls, M.A., and Robert D. Kirk, Jr., M.Ed., my early colleagues in the field; Dr. T. Walter Carlin, Ithaca College, Dr. Thomas A. Mullin, Florida Technological University, Hope Wanderman, M.A., Dr. Ray C. Wunderlich, Pediatrician, and Dr. Andrew D. Holt, President Emeritus, University of Tennessee for their help and encouragement; Chris A. Hawrylak, M.S., for her help in the research for this manuscript; and I wish to thank my father, Nelson T. Barr, for his expert editing, wise counsel and steady encouragement in this and all my projects.

A major portion of the Second Edition is based on the author's doctoral thesis completed while a research scholar in linguistics at Patna University, India, under the supervision of Prof. D. N. Sharma, Vice-Chancellor. Prof. Sharma is a rare individual in whom is combined the best of both the Eastern and Western cultures. It is with the greatest pleasure that this author expresses his profound gratitude to him. My thanks is extended to Vijayshil Gautam, Mrs. Kusum Sharma, Dr. Dipti Tripathi and Dr. N. K. Misra for seeing to my every need while a student in Patna. Thanks is also extended to Dr. S. P. Sinha and Dr. R. P. N. Singh, Patna Medical College, and Dr. V. N. Mishra, Banaras Hindi University, for their help and encouragement.

D.F.B.

CONTENTS

AUDITORY PERCEPTUAL
DISORDERS

CHAPTER 1

INTRODUCTION

The word, even the most contradictory word, preserves
contact—it is silence which isolates.
—Thomas Mann, The Magic Mountain

IT is a generally recognized phenomenon that there are children with both normal intelligence and hearing acuity who have difficulty discriminating among and interpreting auditory stimuli. Such children are said to have an auditory perceptual handicap. They may find it difficult to (1) localize the source of sound, (2) comprehend the meaning of environmental sounds, (3) discriminate among sounds and words, (4) reproduce the pitch, rhythm and melody of music, (5) distinguish and select the significant or important from other sounds, or (6) in speech to combine syllables to form words and words to make sentences.

For lack of suitable research methods, it is difficult to ascertain exactly how such children use their auditory and linguistic listening experience in the course of their development. Assessment of their auditory perceptual problems must too often await the onset of expressive difficulties in speech, reading, spelling and writing.

For present purposes perception may be defined as receiving, processing and classifying sensory information for coding into familiar symbols. Action taken on this input can be immediate or delayed. The most important consideration is how well the child analyzes the input and encodes it into readily understandable symbols so that his attention and energies are free to concentrate on and consider the abstract information thus symbolized. But should the child have perceptual dysfunction, he will exhibit difficulty in his ability to decode, arrange systematically and encode sensory information received. In his dilemma he may strive harder to overcome the handicap, resorting to easily recognizable physical and/or psychological adaptations for this purpose. Or, as the alternative, he may simply avoid the task and thereby fail to

perform at the academic level prescribed for his mental and
chronological age.

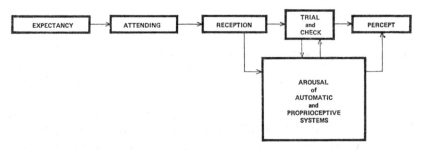

Figure 1. A perceptual model. (Excerpted from p. 18 of *Development of the
Perceptual World* by Charles M. Solley and Gardner Murphy. Basic Books, Inc.,
Publishers, New York, 1960.)

In trying to clarify the perceptual process, Solley and Murphy
(1960) have proposed a perceptual model (see Fig. 1). This model
includes five stages: (1) perceptual expectancy, (2) attending, (3)
reception, (4) trial and check, and (5) final perceptual organization. The model also embodies the autonomic and proprioceptive
arousal system which may exert a degree of control over some
forms of perceptual behavior.

Expectancy. The first component of the model illustrates the
ability to predict the probability of a stimulus occurring with or
following other stimuli. Since our senses are constantly being
animated by stimuli, we need to learn to anticipate what is likely
to occur next so as to integrate effectively stimuli emanating from
the senses.

Attention. Our expectancy of a given stimulus to occur in a
certain pattern motivates us to wait or search for it. Our attention
thus serves to increase the likelihood of our perceiving specific
stimuli. We increase the probability of perceiving a certain plexus
of stimuli from others by the degree of importance we attach to the
given plexus. This is not to say we shut out others altogether, but
rather that we concentrate on the most important plexus at the
moment.

Reception. At this third stage of the perceptual model the nature of the stimulation in relation to our previous experience is of

great importance. If the receptive process is underdeveloped or impaired, we develop our perceptions based on faulty or incomplete information. This results in incorrect meanings being attributed to perceived stimuli.

Trial and Check. At this stage a two-phase process occurs. The expected perceptual pattern is compared with the pattern actually received. In the check phase the tentative preception is then either accepted as empirically valid or invalid. If the prediction concurs with the perceived pattern, we can attribute meaning to it. The amount of trial and check necessary depends on how predictable an event is. If, for example, the redundancy of the stimulus is high, trial and check are but cursory. Thus, trial and check allow us to decode correctly or at least approximately the message contained in a stimulus plexus, thereby affecting its final definition as a valid percept.

VISUAL AND AUDITORY DIFFERENCES

It is important at the outset to understand the main difference between visual and auditory perception. Friedlander (1970) feels that it is a serious mistake to employ models of visual perception research in studying the development of auditory and receptive language. Some reasons are as follows:

1. Incidence. Auditory language disabilities are far more widely distributed among children than are visual perceptual disabilities. Friedlander (1970) mentions a study of children in the special education section of the Madison, Wisconsin, Public School System for the years 1966 and 1967. This system served 2,312 students, and of this total only fourteen children had problems that were specifically visual in nature while 1,050 children had problems related to hearing and language.

2. Research techniques based on visual perception and development do not make major contributions to basic or applied research in the auditory language area; thus, new research models are needed.

3. Obvious differences lie between photic and acoustical energy and between the spatial and temporal domains of vision and hearing.

4. The capacity for listening is accompanied by the capacity to make sounds. This ability to generate stimuli in the same modality as reception has no counterpart in visual experience. This would lead us to conceive of visual and auditory perception as separate information-processing operations, both within the central nervous system and in the course of behavioral adaptation to the environment.

5. The infant's ability to generate self-stimulating prelinguistic and speech sounds plays a unique role in organizing input and monitoring output. This self-generating auditory experience has no counterpart in visual experience. Friedlander (1970) remarks, "To find an analogue in visual perception, one would have to consider the necessity for drawing a picture in order to be able to perceive the important features of a landscape or any other scene."

6. All verbal language perception involves a two-stage perception process since it involves both the discrimination of the basic acoustical properties of the stimulus and the learning of what they stand for. However, most of the visual perceptual experience of the infant or young child is a one-stage process having nonsymbolic, intrinsic significance. It is apparent that most eighteen-month-old children can follow the simple command, "Jane, please bring mother her book." By performing the command, Jane has perceived the symbolic significance of the verbal message and has performed a two-stage symbolic language manipulation she will be unable to perform with abstract visual symbols (writing) for three or four more years.

7. With visual experiences the child can continually examine and reexamine his environment. But in his auditory world, the infant cannot secure a repetition of what is heard except for those sounds he can produce himself. Auditorily, he must often get the message the first time or lose it. Even if the auditory message is repeated, it is seldom if ever the same. Differences occur in the acoustical properties of the message, the phasing, the context, the ambient noise level, the inflections and intonation of the same speaker, and different speakers repeating the same message.

8. Children who adapt to a bilingual environment perform

the extraordinary feat of developing two entirely different language rule systems at the same time. There appears to be no analogue to bilingualism in another perceptual modality.

THE NEUROENDOCRINE CONTROL
OF AUDITORY PERCEPTION

The relationship between adrenal cortical hormone activity and neural activity has been well established. Henkin (1969, 1970) states that sensory detection and integration are regulated by a complex feedback system involving the interaction of the endocrine and nervous sytems. Auditory detection acuity was measured in twenty-five normal subjects and in eight patients with adrenal cortical insufficiency (Henkin, et al., 1967). The patients with untreated adrenal cortical insufficiency exhibited an increased detection threshold for sinusoidal signals by at least 13 dB, particularly between 1000 Hz and 4000 Hz, which is the most sensitive region of human auditory acuity. Treatment with carbohydrate-active steroids alone returned these patients to normal auditory detection-acuity. More importantly, patients with adrenal cortical insufficiency exhibited another type of auditory abnormality, an impairment of integration of auditory information.

One explanation for this integrative defect following removal of carbohydrate-active steroid is that timing of transmission of neural impulses in both the central and peripheral nervous systems is significantly altered. An example of this is difficulty with sound localization. When the sound source is in the midline, localization ability is essentially normal. However, when the sound source is more than 30° from midline, localization ability decreases markedly. Henkin and Daly (1968) feel that these results indicate that it is the temporal factor in sound localization that is critical for these patients. If the sound arrived at the two ears at the same time (if the sound was at midline), these patients could make appropriate judgments of sound azimuth. When, however, the time of arrival of the signal at the two ears is disparate beyond a few milliseconds (when the azimuth is increased to 30° or greater), they were unable to make a correct judgment.

Other integrative difficulty was observed with speech discrimination ability and loudness judgments. The speech discrimination tests were designed to examine another parameter of perceptual or integrative capacity. These patients with untreated adrenal cortical insufficiency exhibited gross impairment in their ability to integrate speech stimuli into meaningful patterns. These untreated patients also noted an increase in harshness or a rasping quality in the tester's voice. This effect can be produced in speech by altering the frequency and intensity relationships or by rapidly switching the signal (altering the temporal relations). Henkin and Daly (1968) suggest that this effect may be the result of a distortion in the patient's appreciation of temporal relationships.

Studies of visual and auditory cortical-evoked potentials in patients with adrenal cortical insufficiency have shown a significant increase in latency of their responses when compared to their latencies after treatment with carbohydrate-active steroids. Feldman et al. (1961) suggest that these disturbances may be due to the direct effect of adrenocortical hormones on the centrally-situated multisynaptic reticular systems of the brainstem which are concerned with the regulation of the electrical activity of the brain as well as with mechanisms of epilepsy, consciousness and mental function.

Henkin (1969, 1970) states that these increases in latency were in the order of 5 to 30 msec and were possibly due to the summation of synaptic delay as the impulse traversed the multisynaptic visual and/or auditory systems. The most marked latency increases (more than 15 msec) occurred in the later or monospecific portions of the evoked response associated with reticular formation activity. Less marked but significant increases in latency (5 to 10 msec) also occurred in the earlier portions of the evoked response. This decrease in conduction velocity across multiple synapses can produce a total decrease in conduction velocity which may be as much as one hundred times slower than in normals.

Henkin (1970) summarizes the effects of carbohydrate-active steroids on normal neural functioning:

> ... for normal sensory function I hypothesize that carbohydrate-active steroids are normally inhibitory, acting as part of a negative feedback system which "inhibits" incoming stimuli. This allows for maximal neural integration of those

stimuli which do reach the central nervous system. Removal of this inhibition results in the functional information loss discussed above. Removal of the inhibition also results in the failure to "shut out" the multiple sensory stimuli to which all of us are constantly exposed. The normal nervous system guards against this occurrence by controlling the level of attention paid to these stimuli partially through the activity of the reticular activation system which in this sense acts as a gain-control mechanism. As shown above, this sytem is particularly sensitive to carbohydrate-active steroid activity.

It is of more than passing interest that associated with the increase in sensory detection acuity after the removal of carbohydrate-active steroid there is a consistent decrease in sensory perception or integration ability. Associated with the decrease in sensory detection acuity which returns to normal after the restitution of carbohydrate-active steroid, there is a consistent increase in sensory perception or integration ability. These phenomena may describe in behavioral terms some important aspects of a general mechanism of nervous sytem function.

These results indicate that carbohydrate-active steroids play a significant role in the manner in which sensation and perception occur. In normal persons these steroids act in an inhibitory manner in both the peripheral and central nervous systems. Their presence inhibits both the detection and perception of sensory input. Their removal releases this inhibition, and sensory detection and perception change dramatically as described in patients with adrenal cortical insufficiency. It appears that reciprocal changes in detection acuity and perceptual ability are related in such a manner that increases in detection acuity are always associated with decreases in perceptual ability. Henkin (1970) feels that this may well be a fundamental concept which relates the manner by which the nervous system detects and processes sensory information of many types. These studies demonstrate and confirm the hypothesis that sensory detection and perception are regulated by a complex feedback system involving the interaction of the endocrine and the nervous system.

In a comprehensive article on adrenal hormones and behavior, Broverman et al. (1974) hypothesize the existence of a central adrenergic-cholinergic balance in favor of adrenergic dominance to enhance performance of serially repetitive tasks and impair performances on perceptual restructuring tasks, while a balance in favor of cholinergic dominance is seen to impair performances of serially repetitive tasks and enhance performances on perceptual restructuring tasks. This implies the existence of antagonism between central adrenergic (sympathetic) and central cholinergic (parasympathetic) neural processes.

The gonadal steroid hormones (estrogen and testosterone) tend to maintain monoamine oxidase (MAO) at intermediate levels of activity that are associated with optimal central adrenergic functioning while the carbohydrate-active (adrenal) steroids are believed to induce a lower level of MAO activity. Long-term stress interferes with estrogen and testosterone production, thereby allowing stress, and induces cortisol to drive the MAO level too low with a resulting accumulation of less efficient *false* neurotransmitters. The false neurotransmitters thus impair central adrenergic functioning, thereby inducing a state of central cholinergic dominance and making the brain less responsive to circulating epinephrine. By administration of gonadal steroids, the physiological and behavioral effects of long-term stress are reversed, allowing for a moderate increase in MAO activity and destruction of the *false* neurotransmitters.

Psychoactive stimulant drugs work by inhibiting monoamine oxidase activity and exert actions across catecholamine-containing nerve terminals. As such they potentiate the availability of the neurotransmitter norepinephrine to the postsynaptic receptors. This permits stimulation of the ascending reticular formation and enhancement of the behavioral reinforcement and short-term memory storage mediated by the limbic system. See Chapters 2 and 3 for discussions on neural transmission, the reticular formation and the limbic system. Chapter 6 discusses drug therapy briefly.

PERCEPTION: AN INDIAN PERSPECTIVE

When constructing or comparing perceptual models for

research, diagnostic or therapeutic purposes, it is important to consider some ancient Indian theories (dating from approximately 600 B.C.) for validity and to gain as well a balanced historical and philosophical view of this primary process. The theories under discussion are the Vedantic, the Nyaya, the Sankhya and the Jaina.

Datta (1972) discusses in detail the Vedantic psychology of perception (*pratyaksa*) drawn so freely from metaphysics. He assesses the value of Vedantic conceptions found to underlie epistemological conclusions, comparing them critically with the more "scientific" Western theories of perception.

According to the Vedantic theory, the mind (*manas* or *antahkarana*), in perceiving an external object, in effect goes out to it through the operative sense or senses (*indriyas*). Thus, the senses are not thought of simply as passively receiving stimuli radiating from the object but as projecting to the object to absorb them. Hence, the senses serve the mind as conveyors of the stimuli generated by what is being sensed. Datta further observes that followers of Western psychology who consider knowledge as deriving from physiological changes must question how the physical can be transmuted to end in the mental. He explains that in the perceptual process the mental is not the terminus of an antecedent physical process, but rather the mind's activity is omnipresent from the start, though the mind may not always be aware of its participation in the initial stages. Only at the end point of a long, often unconscious process where a percept becomes knowledge does the mind's activity reach this fruition and consummation in such a realization.

Thus, in perception the mind acts prior to sense by preadjusting or focusing attention to the object. The mind is thereby directed outside of the organism to the object in space, and in giving attention to the object the mind comes into direct contact with the object. Datta feels that knowledge of the external world is explained by the Vedantic view far more simply and easily than the Western theory of perception that the mind does not go out to the object but only receives the stimuli through the senses coming from the object.

In order to support this theory, Datta takes the case of visual perception. He expresses extreme doubt that from the retinal pictures of external objects we could construct the external world of three dimensions. Western psychologists do not convince Datta when they attempt to explain how from the distribution of light and shade in the retinal pictures we obtain, through inference, the three-dimensional world:

> Without previous knowledge of the external, the mere distribution of light and shade or other local signs would remain mere qualities of pictures painted on a level screen. No Herculean effort of inference could make us project our internal precepts into external space and see them in their real order, magnitude and dimensions.

Datta goes on to explain another fascinating aspect of the Vedantic theory of perception. After an object is removed from the sense, we are left solely with the memory of that object, thus we experience perceiving an image apart and distinct from the object which generated it even though the image as a copy may continue to refer to the original object. Now the question arises "How can one have the exact image in mind of the object no longer presented to the sense?" The only reasonable answer, Datta feels, is that there is a certain principle which somehow accurately records the form and nature of the object when presented to the sense, and it is through a reproduction of this record that one's mind can recall the latter object's essential aspects.

At first reading, it might appear that Datta is merely speaking of long-term memory which involves a structural change in the cortical areas and seems to be dependent upon protein metabolism, but this is not the case. He is stating that this recorded image marks the transition of consciousness from pure subjectivity towards objectivity. This concept thus serves as a mediating principle between the physiological and psychological through which the subject comes to know its object.

This perceptual theory can be compared to the theory of Gestalt psychology. It will be remembered that the Gestalt school speaks of physiological Gestalt which consists of the whole form of the object, a whole that is not a compound construction from many separate stimuli but obtained as a whole from the very beginning.

The Vedantists, accordingly, regard the mind (*antahkarana*) as an instrumental and intermediate principle situated midway between the object and the self. The difference between this and Gestalt theory lies in the Vedantic mental mode (*Vrtti*) being regarded as the result of the interaction between the mind and its object. The Gestalt, either in the physiological or psychological view, is not considered to be the result of such interaction.

It is of interest to note that the Veda also concerns itself with proper speech output as well as perceptual input. Ghosh (1938) mentions the fourteen faults of the Vedantic Chant. "Shyness, fear, extreme loudness, indistinctness, undue nasalization, repressed tone, undue cerebralization, nonobservance of the places of articulation (in general) and (proper) accent, and harshness, creating undue separation between words, uneven tone, hastiness and want of due palatalization." Cautions as to proper recitation include not reciting in an undertone between one's teeth, quickly, haltingly, slowly, with a hoarse voice, in a sing-song manner with repressed voice, omitting (occasionally) words and syllables, and chanting in a plaintive voice. Clearly the Vedantic school was very concerned with proper auditory perception while listening to the Vedantic chant.

According to the Nyaya theory of knowledge, ordinary perception is classified into three modes — *nirvikalpaka* or the indeterminate, *savikalpaka* or the determinate, and *pratyabhijna* or recognition. The first, or *nirvikalpaka*, is limited cognition of the mere existence of an object without any explicit recognition and characterization of it. Prior to discrimination there cannot be any true cognition of an object as a determinate reality. The second, or *savikalpaka*, is perception in which an object is judged as a particular kind of thing. It is determined by certain qualities and is distinguishable from different objects. The process of development from the first modes to the second can be explained by applying association and memory to the cognitive act. The third, or *pratyabhijna*, is the conscious reference of a past and present cognition to the same object (Chatterjee and Datta, 1968; Chatterjee, 1965).

The Sankhya theory of knowledge accepts only three independent sources of valid knowledge (*pramana*) — perception, inference and scriptural testimony (*sabda*). Perception is defined as the direct cognition of an object through its contact with some sense. Both the *nirvikalpaka* and *savikalpaka* modes are accepted as valid and necessary modes of perceptual knowledge. The first arises from the initial moment of contact between a sense and its object. The second mode results from the analysis, synthesis and interpretation of sense-data by the mind or *manas*. Concerning the nature of perception, the Sankhya holds that an object produces certain impressions or modifications in the sense organ. These impressions are analyzed and synthesized by the mind. Through this activity of the senses and the mind, *buddhi* or the intellect becomes modified and transformed into the shape of the object. The intellect reflects, like a transparent mirror, the consciousness of the self (purusa). With the reflection of the self's consciousness in it, the unconscious modification of the intellect into the form of the object becomes illumined into a conscious state of perception (Chatterjee and Datta, 1968).

The Jaina theory recognizes two kinds of ordinary knowledge — *mati* or any kind of knowledge which is ordinary immediate knowledge (or internal and external perception), memory, recognition and inference; and *sruta* or knowledge obtained from authority.

The Jainas give an interesting account of the process by which ordinary perception occurs and is retained. A distinct sensation such as a sound is heard, but its meaning is not yet known. This primary state of conscious awareness is called *avagraha* (or grasping the object). When the question arises as to what the sound is, this state is called *iha* (or query). When a definite judgment is made as to the exact source of the sound, the state is called *avava* (or removal of doubt). Then what has been ascertained concerning the sound is retained in the mind, and this state of retention is called *dharana* (or holding in the mind).

Sruta, the second type of ordinary knowledge, is interpreted as the knowledge obtained from spoken or written authority, i.e. knowledge from what is said or written by others. Since this knowledge is dependent upon auditory and visual perception as well as perception of written letters, *sruta* is said to be preceded by *mati.*

It is interesting to contrast these ancient Indian theories with two current theories of perception. Broadbent (1958) believes that perception is a product of the functioning of a selective filter which can be "tuned" to any one of a number of sources of information available to an individual. This filter discriminates among inputs on the basis of intensity, pitch and spatial localization. Coincidentally, it prevents the overloading of the limited-capacity decision-making system which processes the incoming information and activates the responsible systems and/or stores relevant long-term memory information. Physiologically his model has merit in that the "selective filter" idea parallels the functions of the sensory end organs, the brain stem (particularly the reticular formation and the limbic system), and the terminal cortical areas. The main distinction between Broadbent's model and the Vedantic view is that he describes the perceiver as active only in the sense that certain aspects of available input are accepted and others are blocked out or attenuated. The Vedantic theory attributes a far more active role to the perceiver as the sense goes out to the object and the mind assumes the form of the object perceived.

Another current theory allows for a more active role with the perceiver actually restructuring the input, but still not allowing for as much activity on the part of the perceiver as the Vedantic view. This theory is the concept of analysis-by-synthesis (Stevens and Halle, 1967). According to this theory the perception of auditory stimuli depends on internal generation and matching rather than a simple form of association between perceived stimuli and stored patterns. Normal speech perception can thus proceed only through active participation of the listener whereby hypotheses are formed on the basis of direct analysis and contextual information. They are then verified through an internal replication and matching operation.

A complete comparative study of contemporary perceptual theories or an in-depth philosophical discussion of mind, either as a theoretical construct or as a physiological locus, is within the scope of this paper. The author is attempting, however, in this brief historical discussion of Indian perceptual theories, however limited appears their scientific basis from the West's viewpoint, to orient his thinking somewhat for a greater appreciation of the East's views in this area. From this we in the West may receive a flow of new solutions and clearer, more comprehensive perceptual models upon which to base more definitive research. We should never delude ourselves into believing that Western science has all the answers or even the best approaches to obtain the answers. A looking back or elsewhere to go forward is now an indicated and challenging consideration for expanding the field of our research.

The West tends to accept as valid only those findings and conclusions from logic and other reasoning processes which are largely limited in their application to what is physical and susceptible to direct observation and experimentation.

The East, however, has broadened the uses of the intellect to include study and contemplation of the metaphysical as well, thus deriving wisdom and inspiration from what is evidential but not always demonstrable in human experience. The West objects that what is inferred from the evidential as metaphysical findings is hardly susceptible to proof. The East replies that even circumstantial evidence adduced in her less restricted reasoning techniques is "still very strong, as Thoreau said when he found a trout in the milk jug."

Thus, the idea of the sense acting as a vehicle moving towards the object and not merely a passive receiver of stimuli may appear, on second thought, not so naive or untenable. Likewise, the conception of sense being composed of the same material as the quality of which it can sense would point to a kinship of our physical being to the external world and the consequent fitness of it as a medium for receiving information of the external world.

This author is primarily concerned with how auditory stimuli are received and acted upon in the brain, the emphasis being placed mostly on listening (input) instead of on expression (output). As a result, hearing acuity as an end-organ function is not considered while full attention has been given to auditory reception as a psycholinguistic function. This in turn requires discussion of the nature and extent of auditory perceptual handicaps with therapeutic approaches for their remediation.

Chapter 2

RECEPTIVE FUNCTIONS OF HEARING:
REFLEXIVE AND COMPREHENDING

NERVE impulses are transmitted almost instantaneously by chains of highly specialized cells called neurons in all multicellular animals. Although the physiological time spans over which the communication of metabolic information is relevant are much shorter than the evolutionary periods through which the communication of genetic information extends, these physiological time spans still last over hours, days or weeks. In order to stay alive, however, most animals must respond to certain events in their environment within time spans of seconds or even milliseconds. And since the diffusion of a molecule such as glucose through the space occupied by the cell complex that makes up even so small an animal as a fly requires a few hours, animals must have for survival communication channels that are far faster than those provided by hormones. These high speed channels are provided by neurons. The biological function for communicating neuronal information which neurons form is to generate the rapid stimulus-response reactions that comprise the animal's behavior. Neurons are endowed with two exceptional features that make them apt for this purpose. First, unlike most other cell types, they possess relatively long, thin extensions called axons. With their axons neurons reach and come into contact with the branch-like dendrites of contiguous neurons and, progressively, those at more distant sites. In this way they form an interconnected network extending over the entire animal body. Second, unlike most other cell types, neurons give rise to electrical signals or nerve impulses in response to physical or chemical stimuli. They in turn conduct these signals along their axons and transmit them to other neurons with which they are in contact. The interconnected network of neurons and its traffic of electrical signals form the nervous system.

The nervous system is divided into three parts — (1) an input or sensory part that informs the organism about its condition respecting the state of its external and internal environment; (2) an output or effector part that produces motion by commanding muscle contraction, and (3) an internuncial part (from the Latin *nuncius*, meaning messenger) that connects the sensory and effector parts. The most elaborate portion of the internuncial part, concentrated in the head, is the brain stem and brain.

The processing of data by the internuncial part consists mainly in abstracting the vast amount of data continuously gathered by the sensory organs. This abstraction results from selective destruction of portions of the input data in order to transform residual data into manageable categories that are meaningful to the organism. It should be noted that the particular command pattern issued to the muscles by the internuncial parts depends not only on here-and-now sensory inputs but also on the history of past inputs. Stated more simply, neurons can learn from their own experience.

A brief discussion of how electrical signals arise and travel in the nervous system is important. Neurons, like nearly all other cells, maintain a difference in electronic potential of about a tenth of a volt across their cell membranes. This potential difference arises from the unequal distribution of the three most abundant inorganic ions of living tissue, sodium $(Na+)$, potassium $(K+)$ and chlorine $(CL-)$, between the inside of the cell and the outside, and from the low and unequal specific permeability of the cell membrane to the diffusion of these ions. In response to physical or chemical stimulation the cell membrane of a neuron may increase or decrease one or another of these specific ion permeabilities, which usually results in a shift in the electronic potential across the membrane. One of the most important of these changes in ion permeability is responsible for the action potential, or nerve impulse. Here there is a rather broad but transient change in the membrane potential lasting for only one or two milliseconds once a prior shift in the potential has exceeded a certain much lower threshold value. Thanks mainly to its capacity for generating such impulses, the neuron (a very poor conductor of electric current compared to an insulated copper wire) can carry electrical signals throughout the body of an animal whose dimensions are of the order of inches or feet. The transient change in membrane potential set off by the impulse is propagated with undiminished intensity along the thin axons. Thus, the basic element of signaling in the nervous sytem is the nerve impulse, and the information transmitted by an axon is encoded in the frequency with which impulses propagate along it.

The point at which two neurons come into functional contact is called a synapse. Here the impulse signals arriving at the axon terminal of the presynaptic neuron are transferred to the branch-like dendrite of the postsynaptic neuron that is to receive them. The transfer is mediated not by direct electrical conduction but by diffusion of a chemical molecule, the transmitter, across the narrow gap that separates the presynaptic axon terminal from the dendritic membrane of the postsynaptic cell. That is to say, the arrival of each impulse at the presynaptic axon terminal causes the release there of a small quantity of the chemical transmitter which reaches the postsynaptic dendritic membrane and induces a transient change in its ion permeability. Depending on the chemical identity of the transmitter and the nature of its interaction with the postsynaptic membrane, the permeability change may have one of two diametrically opposite results. On the one hand it may increase the chance that there will arise an impulse in the postsynaptic cell. In that case the synapse is said to be excitatory. On the other hand, it may reduce that chance, in which case the synapse is said to be inhibitory. Most neurons of the internuncial part receive synaptic contacts from not just one but many different presynaptic neurons, some axon terminals providing excitatory and others inhibitory inputs. Hence, the frequency with which impulses arise in any postsynaptic neuron reflects an ongoing process of summation, or, more exactly, a temporal integration of the ensemble of its synaptic inputs.

In lower mammals hearing is mainly a protective sense. Their hearing is the reflexive type developed for instant localization and reaction to sound. Coordination and control of auditory reflex action occur in various centers of the brain stem. The auditory pathway (Fig. 2) shows the centers involved.

In man's evolutionary development, the brain (cortex)

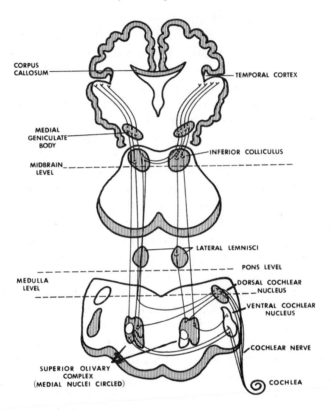

Figure 2. Auditory pathway. Neural connections are shown for only one cochlea, but they are the same for both.

expanded greatly and provided a vast storage area for information from the sensory end organs. Association areas correlated to all the sensory sources of information were also developed. With this increase in the areas of auditory reception, i.e. convolutions of the temporal lobe, man could not only react reflexively to sound, but could recognize, interpret and associate it with various meanings. Thus, another type of *hearing* emerged — comprehending hearing. With man's development of comprehension came his development of speech.

Reflexive hearing is, therefore, basically protective and brain stem coordinated and controlled. Examples of reflexive hearing in infants are the cochleopalpebral reflex (eye-blink), Moro's reflex (contraction of limbs and neck muscles), and increased or decreased heart rate in response to loud sound.

Comprehending hearing is a learned process and occurs only in man. In comprehending hearing, the cortex dominates responses to auditory stimuli instead of the brain stem. The most important auditory stimulus is speech. The infant does not startle reflexively to speech sounds, but attempts to imitate the sounds.

Whitehead (1929), in considering the tasks of infancy, points out that some of the hardest must come first because they are essential to life. He specifically mentions the infant's task of acquiring spoken language with these words:

> The first intellectual task which confronts an infant is the acquirement of spoken language. What an appalling task, the correlation of meanings with sounds! We all know that the infant does it, and that the miracle of his achievement is explicable. But so are all miracles, and yet to the wise they remain miracles.

Friedlander (1969a) points out that normal babies make selective responses to fine auditory signal differences from the very beginning of life if their environment is structured to give their discrimination ability a chance to operate. The infant becomes more and more secure in monitoring environmental sounds with his increased capacity to make more selective responses to fine auditory signal differences. The infant's observation of and attention to his environment constitutes an active, critical and evaluative process characterized by creative model-building and the formation of hypotheses as to what is likely to occur next. These expectancies are formed, then confirmed or rejected by the infant's new experiences. Sanders (1971) describes the infant's perception in this way:

> Initially, the infant recognizes the stimulus complex by its gestalt, without awareness of its components. He is aware of new stimulus complexes by what they are not rather than by what they are, and then later by their overall pattern rather than by their specific components.

For a comparison of the normal child's listening behavior and expressive progress at successive periods from birth to age five years, see Table I.

TABLE I

AUDITORY DEVELOPMENTAL NORMS*
(BIRTH TO FIVE YEARS)

Age	Listening (Receptive) Behavior	Expressive Behavior
Birth thru 4 weeks	1. Responds "reflexively" (startle reactions) to loud environmental sounds. Gross motor reactions to low frequency sounds and "freezing" reactions to high frequency sounds are characteristic. 2. Is quietened by mother's voice when picked up. 3. Diminished activity while attending to a ringing bell.	1. Cry (most characteristic acoustic emission of the infant). 2. Scream. 3. Burp. 4. Vomit sound. 5. Puckering lip sound. 6. Gulp. 7. "Laa" sound. 8. Breath sound. 9. Sneeze. 10. Cough. 11. Gurgle. 12. Whine. 13. Squeak. 14. Whimper.
1 Month	1. Responds to speech. 2. Listens to soft bell sounds and music. 3. Smiles to sound of mother's voice.	1. Makes murmured sounds. 2. Begins vocalizations; cooing, gurgling and grunting sounds.
4 Months	1. Anticipates sounds associated with feeding. 2. Obviously enjoys the sound of noisemakers (rattles, bells). 3. Searches for sound source with eye movements.	1. More substantial cooing, grunting and gurgling. 2. Laughs aloud.
7 Months	1. Bangs rattle, shakes and rings bell with delight. 2. Searches for sound source with head movements. 3. Stops crying on hearing music. 4. Pays attention to speech of the family and responds to angry and pleasant speech. 5. More concerned with tones of voice and inflections than with words.	1. Begins vocalization of "m-m-m" sound while crying. 2. Makes vowel sounds "ah" and "eh." 3. Babbles to persons.

*Modified from Gesell and Amatruda (1967).

Age	Listening (Receptive) Behavior	Sound and Language Development
10 Months	1. Responds to name. 2. Listens to a tuning fork, conversation and to a watch ticking. 3. Listens to and imitates simple sounds. 4. Comprehends "no-no." 5. Responds to verbal request with an action response, e.g. opens mouth when asked.	1. Vocalizes "dada" and "mama" sounds. 2. Uses babbled phrases of four syllables or more. 3. Uses singing tones.
1 Year	1. Gives up his toys on request. 2. Listens with understanding to words. 3. Understands action words and responds in action to commands.	1. Knows and says "mama" and "dada." 2. Begins expressive jargon. 3. Says one or two words clearly.
15 Months	1. Shows shoe on request. 2. Shakes head for "no." 3. Reacts vocally to music. 4. Understands simple questions.	1. Vocalizes wants. 2. Says three to five words meaningfully. 3. Uses short meaningful babble-like sentences (jargon). 4. Babbles monologue when alone. 5. Attempts new words.
18 Months	1. Listens to rhymes, songs, and interesting repetitions of sounds for two to three minutes. 2. Carries out two or more simple directions ("Give it to mother"). 3. Recognizes names of many family members, objects, persons and pets.	1. Says own name. 2. Identifies one common object in a picture. 3. Says ten words. 4. Uses two-word phrases.
2 Years	1. Listens to simple stories. 2. Responds to "Show me a dog, a man, a hat." 3. Points to eyes, ears, mouth upon request. 4. Carries out four or more simple directions.	1. Begins to use three-word sentences. 2. Refers to self by name. 3. Vocabulary of three hundred words. 4. Uses nouns, verbs, and some pronouns.
4 Years	1. Comprehends the meaning of	1. Begins to name at least one

Age	Listening (Receptive) Behavior	Sound and Language Development
	hungry, thirsty and tired. 2. Understands prepositions: behind, beside, on under, and in front. 3. Follows a two-stage command. 4. Comprehends three questions. 5. Recalls a nonsense syllable after thirty seconds.	color correctly. 2. Repeats four digits. 3. Counts three objects by pointing. 4. Uses complete sentences. 5. Vocabulary of 1500 words. 6. Has four-word responses.
5 Years	1. Follows a three-stage command. 2. Recalls a nonsense syllable after forty-five seconds. 3. Can repeat four or five nonsense syllables. 4. Singles out one word to ask its meaning whereas formerly reacted to sentence as a whole.	1. Names five primary colors. 2. Counts ten objects correctly. 3. Names basic coins: pennies, nickels, dimes. 4. Begins to ask the meaning of words and situations. 5. Uses all parts of speech correctly. 6. Uses all consonant sounds. 7. Corrects own errors in learning to pronounce new words. 8. Has number concept of three or four. 9. Vocabulary of 2000 words.

HEARING AND SPEECH DEVELOPMENT

It is a simple rule that sensory input precedes output. Therefore, the organization of effective listening (reception) is imperative for the development of competent speech and language. We know that Friedlander's results (1969b) with infant's selection of vocal reinforcement indicate that the infant's capacity to differentiate auditory signals is far more advanced than his ability to respond.

Friedlander collected data on the listening preferences of infants with automated playtest toys attached to the infant's cribs in their homes. The playtest consists of two large response switches the child can manipulate at will, a loudspeaker, an electrical control and response recorder, and a stereo tape player with a preprogrammed selection of two-channel audio tapes. Whenever the infant operates either switch he automatically records the frequency and duration of his responses and simultaneously turns on one or the other audio tape channels. The two audio channels can be programmed separately for different stimulus materials which contain those variables under investigation. The infant's listening preferences and discriminations are indicated by responses on the switches over an extended period.

The infants, ranging in age from eleven to fifteen months, did

TABLE II

LEVELS OF AUDITORY EXPERIENCE

1. *Primitive awareness.* The background sounds (ambient noise level) of our environment are constantly changing and we are always subconsciously prepared to react to or ignore them. Through this subconscious monitoring of our environment, we are continually aware that we are alive; we subconsciously identify with and become one with our environment.*

2. *Concreteness.* All objects have a "sound-language." That is, objects in their various physical states have the propensity to make certain sounds when moved, banged, felt, kicked, dropped. Therefore, through conscious experience with the sound objects make we later recognize their sounds subconsciously through our auditory memory of them. From this heard-seen-felt perception of objects, we develop concepts of dimension, shape, volume, texture, density, weight, position, relationship of one object to another, and function.

3. *Sensation.* Actual activation of sensori-neural structures by sound.

4. *Perception.* Ability to differentiate among auditory stimuli, according to frequency (pitch), intensity (loudness), harmonics (overtones), for coding into familiar symbols.

5. *Imagery.* Perception and use of objects and sounds around us for our own benefit, as well as remembering their usefulness, value or danger to us.

6. *Arbitrary symbols.* Basic awareness of words as symbols capable of graphic representation.

7. *Symbolic behavior.* Higher symbolic functioning with connotation being applied to symbols (words spoken or written). By connotation is meant the ability to impart representativeness whereby symbols stand for much more than mere graphic representations. Denotation, which is the relation of a symbol to its object, enters in here also.

8. *Conceptualization.* The highest form of awareness characterized by abstract reasoning: that ability to classify and codify into meaningful categories and subcategories to set up an experiential frame of reference which relieves us of the need to experience the same thing repeatedly in order to know it. This backlog of experiential information also serves as a reference point for the transformation and transmutation of learned experience into unique creative forms.

---

*Galambos (1944) reports that there is a spontaneous discharge by ganglion cells, even in the absence of excitation. In his discussion of the spontaneous activity in auditory nerve fibers in particular, he believes that this spontaneous rhythm is the background against which the effects of stimulation are displayed, and by a comparison of the effects against the background, the individual is able to discriminate sound.

not all prefer their mothers' voices. One twelve-month infant in particular preferred to listen to a stranger's lively, well-modulated speech instead of his own mother speaking in a dull, flat monotone. Another infant was offered a choice between two types of his mother's voice, one reproducing her familiar words cheerfully spoken, the other reproducing her voice speaking strange words in a dull, flat tone. As we might anticipate, the infant at first chose the natural mode of his mother's voice, then his preference shifted to her less animated and strange delivery. It is hard to escape the conclusion that these and the other infants studied show a high level of perceptual-cognitive capability for discriminating among the acoustical properties of speech and for subconsciously arranging and rearranging the components of linguistic models as to what is likely to occur next in the presence of familiar or recurrent inputs. Eight levels of auditory experience are explained in Table II.

Normal hearing implies not only a normal auditory mechanism (external, middle, inner and central auditory areas), but the ability to understand the sounds heard. See Figure 3 for the basic anatomy of the auditory mechanism. Speech is complex sound in which many frequencies are present at various intensities; therefore, sufficient vowel consonant combinations must be under-

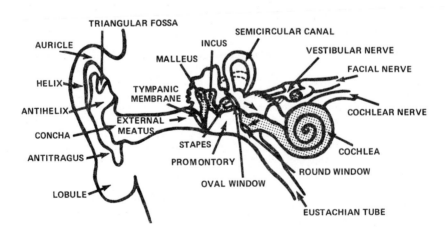

Figure 3. The basic anatomy of the auditory mechanism.

stood at a proper intensity level (usually 40 to 60 dB above threshold) for correct interpretation of words and sentences to occur. (See Table III for speech sound developmental norms.)

TABLE III

SPEECH SOUND DEVELOPMENTAL NORMS*

Sound	Initial	Medial	Final	Sound	Initial	Medial	Final
By Age 3½				*By Age 5½*			
p	pie	happy	cup	f	four	coffee	off
b	boy	table	tub				
m	milk	hammer	home	*By Age 6½*			
w	wet	away	—	v	very	river	five
h	hand	behave	—	th	that	mother	bathe
				sh	shoe	ocean	fish
By Age 4½				ch	chin	teacher	match
				j	joke	pigeon	orange
d	dog	lady	bed	l	lady	balloon	ball
t	tie	potato	cat				
n	nose	funny	run	*By Age 7½*			
ng	—	finger	ring	s	soup	inside	ice
g	gum	wagon	egg	z	zipper	easy	ears
k	key	bacon	book	r	red	carry	car
y	yes	onion	—	th	thumb	bathrub	teeth

*Modified from Poole (1934).

SOME VARIABLES OF AUDITORY RECEPTION

It is important at this point to look at some of those variables which affect receptive language processes:

Variables of Signal and Message*

First is the variable of *stimulus selection*. This is the recognition and selection problem facing the young child attending speech in his natural environment which is embedded in various intensity levels, high ambient noise, varying rapidity of the

*Modified from Friedlander (1970).

speech stream, incomplete and distorted grammatical structures, and two or more people speaking at once. Second is the variable of *recurrence*. When considering the absence of recurrence in auditory and language perception, it is clear that vision is different from audition when attempting to construct a perceptual and organizational learning model. With vision the child can continually examine and reexamine his spatial environment. Through this constant accessible visual stimulation the child acquires concepts of form, space, shape, color, and so on. In auditory language perception, however, the child rarely has a chance for a repeat performance. Auditorily he must usually get the information when first presented or lose it. The very fact that most children develop normal auditory and language perception attests to the extraordinary ability of the auditory mechanism to discriminate. Third is the variable of *control of expression*. This variable points up the major difference between listening and speaking. If the listener is listening effectively, he is controlled by the receptive process. The speaker, however, controls the expressive process and determines his message content, word order, grammatical structure, rate, intonation and gestures. The listener, therefore, must willingly abandon some self-consciousness to attend the speaker. If he fails to lose himself into complete attentiveness, his communication with the speaker is incomplete. Fourth and last is the variable of *convergence and divergence*. Listening is convergent in that the listener exercises fewer options while attending and reconstructing speech. Speech, however, is less restrained, has unlimited options for expression and sentence generation, and is therefore divergent. It is obvious that if the divergent characteristics of speech prove a mismatch with the convergent characteristics of listening, communication must fail.

The Variable of Physio-Psychological Readiness

The variable reflects the physical and psychological integrity of the organism at a given age. The child is expected to possess the mental capacity and the physiological and psychological maturity to acquire *average* facility with receptive and expressive language. Likewise, the child should have no sensory defect at the end organ of hearing, nor any trauma or injury to the cortical and subcortical areas of the brain. Should injury or defect be present, the questions of extent and area of damage, of nature and degree of hearing loss, and of time of onset become crucial.

Variables of Temporal Dimension

The auditory cues of speech consist of sound sequences where phonemes are arranged and combined to constitute a dynamic language unit. Decoding of these sound sequences becomes possible and is facilitated because of their essential differences in frequency, amplitude and duration. For instance, vowel sequences having similar phonetic properties are distinguished largely by their duration when enunciated, e.g. *ba, va* and *wa*. Discriminations in sound sequences, therefore, can occur due to the rate at which changes occur between the sounds, changes in frequency or intensity, changes in the order of sound sequences, and changes in intonation and rhythmic patterns. Thus, in considering all variables of temporal dimension, time is the critical factor.

Variables of Memory Function

The memory function is crucial to the organization of receptive experience. During this stage of the information-handling process, new inputs are compared with inputs already stored. Without the storage and retrieval process of the short and long-term memory functions, all sounds heard would forever be novel and considered as if received for the first time. There could be no reference to, and comparison with, similar or related sounds previously heard but unavailable for readout.

Variables of Home and Security

The early environmental influences on the infant are of great importance in his formulating a receptive language. The infant's receptive system is malleable and easily shaped during his first few months of life. Important factors in developing his receptivity during this early stage include the degree of parental contact and influence, stimulative effects of the parental speech, order of his birth with respect to siblings and their interrelationships, family size and the presence of lively family members to stimulate and reinforce his urge to partake of the interactions of fellow members and to reciprocate in kind with those in his immediate environment.

CEREBRAL DOMINANCE AND AUDITORY PERCEPTION

Dichotic listening tasks have provided a new technique for the study of cerebral dominance. In dichotic listening situations the listener attends two different auditory signals simultaneously, one at the right ear and one at the left ear. Recent studies have shown functional differences between the two cerebral hemispheres in the perception of verbal and nonverbal stimuli. Verbal signals such as digits and words when presented dichotically are heard better by most subjects at the right ear-left hemisphere (Kimura, 1961, 1967). The opposite — that is, better accuracy at the left ear-right hemisphere — has been found for nonverbal signals such as melodies (Kimura, 1964, 1967), 1000 Hertz pure tones and white noise (Tsunoda, 1969), and environmental sounds (Curry, 1967). It is apparent, therefore, that in dichotic verbal listening both hemispheres receive a stronger signal from the contralateral pathway and a weaker stimulus from the ipsilateral pathway. In terms of figure-ground discrimination this perceptual dominance would allow the stronger signal to be acted upon as the figure while the weaker signal would be inhibited or stored. The dominant hemisphere is, therefore, a better inhibitor of verbal and nonverbal material as well as being a superior perceiver of verbal material (Barr and Carmel, 1970).

As the average child develops, progressive lateralization of language occurs in the left hemisphere, which is independent of handedness. This process generally begins at about two years of age and may be complete at five years of age (Kimura, 1967). However, much functional plasticity of higher nervous system integration is evident up to the age of twelve or thirteen years (Obrador, 1964).

It is obvious that children vary greatly in their development of dominance. Sometimes, such as with some stutterers (Curry and Gregory, 1969) and with certain brain-injured individuals, cerebral dominance for auditory stimuli does not occur. This lack of dominance in both hemispheres often results in a type of cerebral organization open to many forms of perceptual stress (Critchley, 1962).

In a recent study, Ling (1971) presented sequences of digits to nineteen hearing-impaired children and to nineteen normal hearers. The digits were presented both dichotically and monaurally. She found that the normal hearing children were superior to the hearing impaired in the recall of both monaural and dichotic digits. The right ear dichotic scores were superior for the normal-hearing group, but the intersubject variability among the hearing impaired was so great that no right or left ear advantage could be found. No correlation was found between the degree of ear asymmetry on the dichotic test and vocabulary scores for the hearing impaired. Both digits of a dichotic pair were rarely reported by the hearing impaired. Apparently one digit was masked or suppressed by the other. Ling concluded that speech lateralization could not be inferred from dichotic digit scores among hearing-impaired children.

Sklar et al. (1972) collected EEG data on a group of normals and a group of children with reading disorders. The two groups differed in three ways. Less synchronization between the cerebral hemispheres was found among the experimental group with dyslexia, but more synchronization within each hemisphere was in evidence. In general, more theta waves (3 to 7 cycles per second) were present among the reading disabled group. These findings lead Sklar to theorize that reading disorders in children are related to incomplete cerebral dominance. He further points out that increased theta activity is characteristic of people in new and novel environments and speculates that part of the dyslexic's problem is that his world is never quite familiar to him. It remains for future research to establish a possible relationship between increased theta activity and impaired memory ability due to poor synchronization between the hemispheres. Another profitable area of investigation might be the role played by the brain stem (particularly the reticular formation) in this dysynchronization. See Chapter 3 for a discussion of reading problems, the brain stem and the reticular formation. Chapter 4 contains a discussion of the electroencephalogram (EEG) in the diagnoses of minimal brain dysfunction.

Witelson and Pallie (1973) obtained anatomical measurements of the language-mediating area of the superior surface of the temporal lobe (planum temporale) for both the left and right hemispheres for a group of fourteen neonatal and sixteen adult human brain specimens. The left-sided area was found to be statistically significantly larger in the neonate as in the adults. This suggests that anatomical asymmetry is present before any environmental effects such as language learning and unimanual preference and may therefore be an important factor determining the typical pattern of left hemisphere speech lateralization found in most adults. Furthermore, their findings suggest that such neonatal asymmetry indicates that the infant is born with a "preprogrammed biological capacity to process speech sounds."

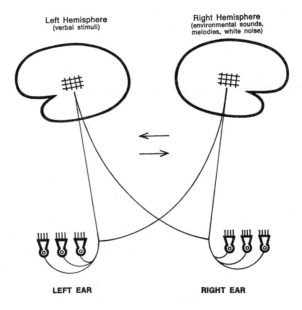

Figure 4. Auditory pathways representing cerebral dominance asymmetries.

Papcun et al. (1974) speculate that the left hemisphere is specialized for processing the sequential parts of which a stimulus is composed. Language is lateralized to the left hemisphere because of its dependence on segmental subparts, and this dependence characterizes language perception as distinct from most other human perception.

Certainly, much more research is needed investigating the nature and extent of dominance difficulties among children with minimal brain dysfunction. Figure 4 depicts the auditory pathways representing cerebral dominance asymmetries.

Chapter 3

AUDITORY PERCEPTUAL DISORDERS

THERE are many names given to describe the etiological factors involved in perceptual disorders: central nervous system dysfunction, CNS maturational delay, minimal brain injury, cerebral dysfunction, psychoneurological learning disability, the dysynchronous child. The term this author chooses to use is *minimal brain dysfunction* due to insufficient functional development resulting in impaired learning and motor abilities. Brain dysfunction is not intended to imply only structural damage but would include maturational delay, biochemical aberrations, endocrine changes, neurohormonal changes and phychoneurological anomalies. The problem, therefore, stems from within the child and is not a result of environmental factors alone.

Wunderlich (1970) speaks of a common denominator in most learning disorders:

> The common denominator in most learning disorders is a developmental fixation at a primitive level of function. This seems to hold true whether the prime problem is brain damage, improper environment, chronic psychic stress, or heredity. Consider the frequent application of the term "immature" to children who have problems in the classroom. This concept of failure to progress beyond certain developmental levels is a useful one and may refer to total overall function or only to an isolated skill.

Often the practitioner is confused from considering the complex symptomatology of children having minimal brain dysfunction. This is because of the many possible, some conflicting, etiologies, all of which, however, can result in inadequate CNS development and functioning.

Genetic Factors

Orton (1937) mentions lineage etiology among children with

34

reading, writing and speech problems. Drew (1956) considers the genetic factor dominant among children with reading disabilities. In his reporting of a chromosonal study, Lenneberg (1967) supports the tendency to have language and learning disabilities run in families. It seems safe to assume that many specific learning disabilities as well as general mental deficiency in many cases are traceable to hereditary factors. Silver (1971) reports that his familial study firmly suggests a genetic factor in MBD. He further suggests that there is evidence of an inherited "type of nervous system" in which the pathology might be due to a neurohumoral imbalance. The frequency with which one finds either siblings with the same types of disabilities or either parent reporting specific learning problems in school has not been overlooked by Silver. He suggests that this familial trait results in a nervous system in which the perceptual, cognitive, memory and/or expressive functions are altered. Studies of this type point out the need for further studies of the genetic aspects of MBD.

Biochemical or Metabolic Factors

Kurtz (1965) lists approximately two hundred metabolic disorders which may result in brain dysfunction. However, McGrady (1968) reports only one percent of the brain-injured are known to exhibit metabolic disorders manifested in neurological, intellectual or behavioral difficulties. He mentions only six such disorders susceptible to such identification: glycinemia, phenylketonuria, histidinemia, homocystinuria, maple syrup urine disease (disorders of amino acid or protein metabolism), and galactosemia (disorder of carbohydrate metabolism).

Maturational Factors

Obviously maturational delay can possibly result in inadequate CNS functioning. Nor is it safe to assume that all children with perceptual problems will spontaneously outgrow their problems without residual language and learning disabilities. In considering maturational factors, Church (1961) cautions that "theories which assume that ontogenetic changes in behavior are produced by maturational changes must take account of the possibility that many maturational changes are in turn induced by perceptual stimulation." He continues by stressing the relationship of maturation to experience in saying, "while some part of the change that occurs in infancy can be accounted for in terms of physical maturation, we know that maturation stands in a circular feedback relationship to experience — the things the organism does, feels, and has done to it."

Trauma or Injury

This etiology would cover brain disorder due to physical injury, often after the brain has achieved some maturity and then is disrupted by the trauma. Trauma might also include anoxia, toxemia which usually causes CNS damage during the prenatal and transnatal stages of development.

Metal Poisoning

Special mention should be made of the problem of neurological impairment due to metal poisoning, resulting in specific learning disabilities and mental retardation. The ingestion of lead-based paints, eating and drinking from cups and plates with a high lead content, and breathing lead-laden air from automobile emissions has added dramatically to the number of perceptually handicapped children, particularly among ghetto children. Here, obviously, is a man-created problem which can be alleviated by removing dangerously high levels of lead from the environment.

Mercury poisoning presents another hazard. Mercury gets into the air, soil and water. Main contributors are chlorine plants pulp and paper mills, paint and refining plants, mining wastes, industrial discharge, fossil fuels, sewage, etc. Mercury apparently seeks out nervous tissues, particularly the brain. This fact explains the bizarre neurological symptoms of spasticity, ataxia, mental retardation, seizures and generalized brain damage.

The possible resulting auditory problems can loosely be divided into receptive and expressive disorders, although both disorders most often exist in combination. It must be remembered that the child with an auditory perceptual handicap hears *normally* sensorywise, but he (1) does not interpret what he hears, (2) does not understand environmental sounds or the spoken word, and/or (3) cannot categorize or structure his auditory world. He therefore responds inconsistently and inappropriately to auditory stimuli.

AUDITORY RECEPTIVE DISORDERS

Children with receptive disorders are often thought to be deaf or hard of hearing due to their inappropriate and inconsistent responses to sound. They tend to fatigue easily in the presence of ambient noise and speech and therefore tend to become frustrated quickly in conversational situations. This auditory *overloading* results also in an abnormally short attention span in that these children become distracted easily and lose the auditory message or figure in the ambient noise level.

Some of these children with severe auditory perceptual problems have trouble with exogenous auditory awareness. In this case they direct their attention or awareness inwardly to their own body sounds rather than toward the external sounds of their environment. This form of auditory immaturity can be more easily understood when one considers the confusion these children have when attending sounds in the environment, and the end result of such inward directed awareness is often a poor body image. Auditorily, we may say these children are strangers to their environment. They may realize they are different, that they do not comprehend auditory stimuli as do their peers, and they sometimes retreat inwardly to an auditory world with which they are most familiar — their own bodies.

Rimland (1964) feels that the severe auditory perceptual problems sometimes found in infantile autism and schizophrenia may be the result of reticular formation dysfunction. Their echolalia-type of speech indicates receptive and expressive functioning with little or no integration of meaning. They therefore apprehend but do not comprehend stimuli. Silver (1971) finds many common perceptual and cognitive features in schizophrenia, autism and minimal brain dysfunction. He questions whether or not they are

variations on the same theme, and whether those differences based
on the specific neurohumoral imbalance or on the site of imbalance within the system. Staehelin (1944) postulates a subcortical
dysfunction in *true* schizophrenia. More specific localization of
the dysfunction is thought by Roberts (1963) and Smythies (1966)
to be a disturbance of the limbic system and its diencephalic and
cortical connections, especially the temporal lobe. Rosenzweig
(1955) points to a disturbance of a homeostatic mechanism dependent on a reticular formation-thalamus-cortex circuit. The
limbic system and its relationship to schizophrenia are discussed
in greater detail later on in this chapter.

Often problems with awareness exist because of difficulty in
localizing the source of sound. Any sound that is fifty micro-
seconds out of phase from midline should result in localization
knowledge in the normal child as to the location of the sound
source. Phase (timing of the arrival of sounds) is also important
for the temporal ordering of auditory patterns incident at the
temporal cortex resulting in our ability to discriminate sounds
heard.

Getman (1969) makes the following observations concerning
children with auditory localization difficulties:

> The observations of children who cannot localize a noise
> within an arc of 360 degrees makes them considerably different
> than the subjects who can discriminate changes in the azimuth
> position of as little as one degree from the median plane. Some-
> where in this difference between the beginner and the sophisti-
> cate is the process of learning to localize the noise after having
> learned that all orientations must be made from one's self as the
> zero-point — the ego-centric locus.

He continues by making a connection between visual perceptual problems and auditory localization difficulties.

> All the evidence in visual performance and the accumulating
> evidence in our observations of auditory performance reminded
> us that a child could not consistently identify anything he could
> not localize. If he did not know where a thing was, he could not
> accurately identify it.

With the absence of tactual and visual cues, perception of hori-
zontal direction (azimuth) of the sound source depends upon

differential stimulation of two ears with respect to time and intensity. Localization of sound is thought to occur at the medial geniculate bodies of the brain stem (see Fig. 2).

Rose et al. (1966) found that for tonal stimuli of long duration of the cat, interaural phase differences have been shown to affect markedly the firing of units in the inferior colliculus. This effect could serve to specify differences in time of arrival at the two ears. Thus, "the shape and the extent of the receptive field of a neuron which is sensitive to interaural time differential presumably vary with the range of delays to which the neuron responds." It is important to remember also that intensity differences at the two ears are of great importance, especially for the directional localization of high tonal frequencies.

Auditory discrimination problems consist of (1) synthesis (combining parts of speech to form a whole), (2) sequencing (arranging words in proper order), (3) figure-ground (isolating and discriminating desired sound from background noise), (4) phonemic discrimination (words sounding alike but having different meanings), and (5) auditory integration of words with multiple meanings (to select meaning intended or most appropriate in the context).

AUDITORY PERCEPTION AND READING PROBLEMS

The relationship of auditory perception to reading is well established. Evans (1969) draws the following conclusions concerning auditory and auditory-visual integration skills as they relate to reading: (1) in a developmental sense, the ability to discriminate auditorily may be particularly important in developing the visualized vocabulary; (2) skill in auditory-visual and visual-auditory sensory integrations are positively correlated with reading achievement; (3) poor readers appear to be significantly more impaired in these integrative skills than good readers, even when the two groups are equal in auditory memory, visual and auditory discrimination, and IQ's; and (4) enough evidence appears to exist to warrant attention to auditory functions in preparatory or remedial reading classes.

Wunderlich (1970) describes the process of learning to read in this way:

> Learning to read is a decoding process. The child must learn
> to know that thoughts and meanings are derived from aggre-
> gates of symbols which have meaning only by virtue of prior
> agreement among the makers of the symbols. Immediately we
> can see that the child is dealing in the world of symbol manipu-
> lation for purposes of information and communication. If he
> has no need to decipher the code, he will not; if he has channels
> of communication open to him that provide all his information
> and communication needs, he will have no reason to learn to
> decipher the code; if he has handicaps in interpreting incoming
> sensory information or in central integration of the informa-
> tion, he may feel that the code is not worth the effort, especially
> if the child is not supported by those authority figures around
> him who must say, in essence, "it *is* worthwhile to struggle with
> it, Johnny; go ahead, I'll help you and encourage or demand."
> ... The first way parents help is by *talking* so the auditory brain
> can record the register, then so the child can mimic; the next way
> parents help is by *shutting up* so he can talk.

Luria (1966) found that phonetic and synthesis problems often
result from lesions in the auditory cortex. Often the discrepancy
between true reading ability and the limited ability to recognize a
few printed letters or words is characteristic of children who have
difficulty establishing grapheme-phoneme correspondences due
to temporal lobe dysfunction. In their investigation of the ability
of first grade children to match auditory and visual information,
both inter- and intrasensorywise, Muehl and Kremenak (1966)
found that matching visual pairs was easy for most children.
Matching visual to auditory to visual pairs caused an intermediate degree of difficulty. They concluded that the ability to
match visual pairs did not contribute to the prediction of reading
achievement, while the ability to match visual to auditory, auditory to auditory, and auditory to visual pairs made significant
contributions to the prediction of reading achievement. Rosner
and Simon (1970) point out that reading is primarily an
auditorily-based skill and that visual analysis of symbols is less
demanding than the analysis of verbal sounds to the typical first
grade child learning to read.

LANGUAGE LEARNING PROBLEMS

The average child acquires language based upon perceived morphemic and melodic patterns. These perceived patterns are dependent upon a two-fold differentiation on the part of the child — the intonational contour (melody pattern) and the discrimination of syllables, morphemes and morpheme combinations in sequential order. The syllable is the irreducible acoustic unit, with the critical cues being the transitions between phonemes and morphemes (Berry, 1969).

For the child with auditory perceptual dysfunction, language learning often degenerates to learning by adding one sound to another, and so on, in an attempt to perceive meaning. These children lack the ability to use the important cues contained in the transitional phases of sounds. The morpheme is a minimal unit of speech that is both recurrent and meaningful. It may be composed of a word (a free morpheme) or a part of a word (a bound morpheme). The most important fact is that the morphemic unit forms the perceptual basis of sound sequences. Children with auditory perceptual dysfunction do not perceive the acoustic-kinesthetic cues (auditory and movement patterns) occurring as transitional sounds within and between sequences.

Berry (1969) discusses the psycholinguistic components of language — phonology, syntax and semantics.

Phonology is the study of the phonemic and prosodic patterns that comprise the speech event and is a generally-used term describing the speech event itself. Prosody, the musical quality of our speech, is the earliest dimension of phonology to be employed by the infant in his comprehension and use of language. The melody of our speech varies in tonal characteristics due to changes in pitch, quality, loudness and duration. Intonational patterns are first formed by changes in the fundamental frequency or the pitch as the infant cries and breathes. Thus, modification of intonation will occur due to an innately determined organization of the respiratory and phonatory muscles as well as by changes in loudness, duration and frequency stress. Speech rhythm is dependent upon the temporal-spatial patterning of syllables, words and phrases and stress factors. The nuances of one's speech are very much dependent on vocal quality which convey subtle meaning and heighten perceptual cues as rich overtones are developed.

Syntatic Structure. Chomsky (1967) was among the first to point to the universal features of grammar. He believes that these universal rules which generate functional grammars are innate in the human being for they vary little from language to language. It is therefore the task of the linguist to discover these rules.

Children develop word order sense — subject, verb and direct object. Though at eighteen months, children reduce the number of words when imitating adult sentences, they preserve the syntax. They appear to telescope their speech, discounting those syntatic class words that are less important in terms of semantic content. Children by thirty months are well on their way to developing syntatic structure whereby they identify phrase structures, use articles *a, an, the* with noun-phrases, understand the difference between imperative and declarative sentences, and comprehend the multiple meanings of words and make fine contextual discriminations. Children with auditory perceptual dysfunctions often do not perceive those natural phrase structures in the string of words that comprise a sentence, nor do they know noun and verb phrases and which words belong in each class.

Semantics is the perception of linguistic meaning, in particular the relationships of signs to their referents. In early language comprehension the child perceives as a whole the total frame of reference: the background noise, gestures, body postures, facial expressions and contextual cues. Thus, normal children comprehend meaning in terms of complete units (of phrases or sentences). They learn to categorize words and sequences of words and learn the relationships between perceived objects or experiences and their definitive categories. See Chapter 2 for some variables which affect receptive language processes and for the levels of auditory awareness.

The expressive language ability of children with auditory perceptual dysfunction is often limited by problems with parts of speech. Some trouble with nouns is present, but the most trouble is found with words that express action (verbs), quality and feelings (adjectives). The nouns that give most trouble are those that pertain to parts of the body. Dates, time and abstractions are especially difficult. Prepositions which denote relationships, e.g. on, in, under, often cause difficulty.

In considering abstractions, it is important to remember that self and the concept of self are abstractions — to know oneself as an entity separate and unique from the environment is most truly achieved when one knows oneself as auditorily unique. This becomes all the more problematic when we consider that many of these children have auditory feedback difficulties. The information supplied by their hearing is often faulty due to problems with temporal ordering of language patterns. A delay of milliseconds in the temporal ordering of auditory symbols can distort the meaning. Slight alterations in the time sequences or rhythmic patterns can place the auditory impulse out of phase both with auditory impulses and with impulses from other contributing modalities.

THE TEMPORAL LOBE

The temporal lobe appears to be concerned with the interpretation of experience, with certain complex sensory functions, and probably with laying down permanent memory stores. The superior and lateral portions appear to be primarily concerned with sensory function. Stimulation in these areas of conscious subjects leads to interpretative illusions:

a. sounds seem louder or softer, closer or further away, clearer or less distinct
b. visual objects appear larger or smaller, closer or further, clearer or distorted, and their apparent speed of movement may be altered
c. recognition is affected in that present experience may take on a feeling of illusory familiarity (*déjà vu*) or, as the alternative, a familiar scene may become unfamiliar and/or altered in some undefinable way
d. various strong emotions such as fear, sorrow, guilt, disgust and loneliness may appear

Possibly these findings of Penfield and Roberts (1959) indicate that the temporal cortex acts as a sort of fine control over various aspects of audition and vision as well as inducing emotional reactions such as the feeling of familiarity or strangeness that so links perception, emotion and memory. The temporal cortex also appears to act as a detailed memory store where a continuous experiential record of our experiences are stored complete with the emotions we felt at the moment of experience. The temporal lobe also appears to compare present and past experience. See Chapter 2 for a discussion of the temporal lobe and cerebral dominance.

SUBCORTICAL AND CORTICAL SPECIFIC LESIONS

It is extremely difficult to identify clear-cut limited lesions which support theoretical concepts of the types and degree of the resulting language problems. Schuell (1964) has observed that there is a language function per se which is disturbed wherever the lesion is located in the speech and auditory areas of the dominant hemisphere. A common defect is inability to scan memory to recall a word. Clearly then, word patterns are well dispersed over the area of the cortex.

The lesion can be specific as to the area of the cortex involved while being general in the pattern of the resulting language

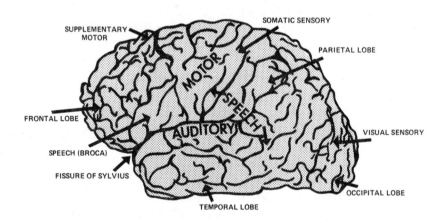

Figure 5. Basic anatomy of the left cerebral hemisphere.

disorder. Some studies of language disorders arising from cortical specific lesions have been made. See Figure 5 for the basic anatomy of the left cerebral hemisphere.

Understanding a simple sentence requires knowledge of grammatical structures, short-term memory storage and the self-control to question premature conclusions. Lesions at the temporal cortex, however, may limit the number of verbal signals processed, thereby suppressing understanding. Left temporal lobe lesions may result in the failure to establish word-name associations for actions, qualities, states of being and the relative importance of considered objects. In these cases the sequence of words is not retained as the length of the series increases. Often, with temporal lobe damage, only a fragment of the sentence is grasped instead of being understood as a whole.

Lesions in the superior temporal lobe region may result in defects of phonemic perception (Luria, 1965). Lesions of the middle portion of the dominant temporal lobe (usually the left) resulted in difficulty in reproducing the sequence of words in their proper order (Luria, 1966). Difficulty in understanding the meaning of a word, even after repetition, has also been found. Apparently the inhibition is augmented by repeated presentations. With lesions of the frontal-temporal lobe regions, Luria (1966) found that the subjects had difficulty in understanding the meanings of abstract words, particularly metaphorical and allegorical meanings as well as difficulty in establishing and reproducing rhythm patterns. Associated lesions of the temporal and occipital lobes have been found by Luria to result in integrative dysfunction in establishing auditory-visual correspondences between objects and their names.

With occipital-parietal lobe lesions, Conrad (1932) found impairment of simultaneous syntheses and orientation in space and difficulty in naming objects and actions. Complex word constructions which can be reversed or transformed, such as active and passive voice, may be affected by integrative dysfunctions of the parieto-occipital systems.

TEMPORAL LOBE EPILEPSY IN CHILDREN

The problem of temporal lobe epilepsy in children has received little attention from educators and pathologists in dealing with the learning child so disabled. This disorder is most easily diagnosed during the course of a seizure by observing the EEG recording of generalized discharges featured by the atypical spike and wave pattern. The seizures are psychomotor. Another diagnostic indicator is a good therapeutic response to an anticonvulsant such as phenytoin or primidone which has little or no general psychological effect.

Incidence

Pond and Bidwell (1960) found that 17 percent of all epileptic children between the ages of ten and fourteen years had temporal lobe epilepsy. Graham and Rutter (1968) found an incidence figure of 13 percent for epileptic children between the ages of five and fourteen years. Both studies show a higher incidence of temporal lobe epilepsy among adults of 26 percent.

Etiology

Etiological factors could be tumors and degenerative lesions (rare in children); know *insults*, e.g. head injury at birth, meningitis or encephalitis; or unclear *insults*. The presence of widespread *patchy* lesions may help to explain several clinical phenomena seen in these children and would account for the accompanying intellectual backwardness commonly associated with these injuries. The more circumscribed the lesion, the better the intelligence (Ounsted et al., 1966). The widespread nature of the neuropathological changes helps to explain the "mixed" seizure pattern and explains why relatively few of these children are fit for temporal lobectomy (Pond, 1969).

Clinical Symptoms

Classical neurological signs such as hemiplegia are only infrequently seen in children with temporal lobe epilepsy.

Children with cerebral palsy have attacks which usually have prominent motor components without typical symptoms of temporal lobe epilepsy. If the neurological symptoms do coexist, the patients have fairly extensive brain damage.

The two most prominent behavioral features are extreme temper tantrums (paroxysmal rage) and hyperkinesis. The author has found that the temper tantrums are not more common in children with low intelligence. The children with hyperkinesis, however, generally are of lower intelligence, with the symptom seen more often in boys than in girls, and is much commoner among those of early age. Hyperkineses in their cases resemble those found in brain-damaged children without epilepsy. The clinical symptoms found by the author are in agreement with those found by Pond et al. (1961).

The rhinencephalic-midbrain complex is the implicated area drawing most research attention. Chronicity is one of the most characteristic features of temporal lobe epilepsy, and it is in contrast to other forms of childhood epilepsy which tend to die out with increased age, and therefore do not contribute to the adult epileptic population.

Drug Therapy

Childhood temporal lobe epilepsy as in adults is relatively resistent to the usual anticonvulsant drugs. Primidone® appears to be the most reliable. Such anticonvulsants have little effect on the behavioral disturbances, however, and a phenothiazine such as chlorpromazine may be of therapeutic value. The usual difficulty here is to steer between oversedation and uncontrolability since the anticonvulsant drugs must be continued while other drugs are being used. A recent hypothesis relating to anticonvulsant medication is the suggestion that many of the chronic psychiatric abnormalities of epileptics, including schizophrenia-like states, are precipitated by a disturbance of vitamin B12 and folic acid metabolism due to prolonged treatment with anticonvulsant drugs (Reynolds et al., 1966, 1967).

The plasticity of the child's brain means great recovery of function can occur, even when comparatively large areas are destroyed. This is particularly true of the neocortex but not so true of the lower level motor cortex areas such as the sensory motor area and the primary occipital visual receiving areas which show little or no recovery of function after even slight lesions (Turner, 1969).

Learning Disturbances

Children with temporal lobe epilepsy suffer more impediment in language-learning ability than those with temporal lobectomies (as measured by the Wechsler Scale). Milner (1958) reports the most marked deficit following left temporal lobectomy was in verbal learning ability. Blakemore (1969) points out that even those with dominant (usually left) temporal lobectomies can enjoy return of verbal language function if instructional material is presented at a slower than normal rate. Good return is usually seen within one year postoperatively.

Severe memory loss can occur, however, if the hippocampus and the amygdala are removed. The difficulty involves poor ability to commit to memory new material and early recall problems with recent memory. Usually associational and remote memory are preserved.

However, functional plasticity of the damaged neocortical areas suggests guarded optimism as far as positive results in verbal language therapy are concerned. There is the distinct possibility of establishing new learning and retention traces in the nervous system following intervention of drug and language therapies. Less plasticity is to be expected in children with temporal lobe epilepsy than with those who have undergone temporal lobectomies.

Clearly the informed educator and/or therapist must consider all aspects of temporal lobe epilepsy in children in formulating adequate programs for educating and rehabilitating such disadvantaged children, taking care to tailor these programs to meet the special needs of each child. This realistic approach to a generally-neglected problem area can prove most effective and rewarding to all concerned.

INTERSENSORY INTEGRATIVE DISORDERS

Some children with perceptive handicaps evidently perceive

normally when receiving stimuli through a single sensory modality. When, however, the perceptual task involves several modalities or multiple stimuli are received through the same modality, breakdown of the receptive system often occurs. Failure of the child's ability to integrate multiple input from two or more sensory modalities is termed an *intersensory integrative disorder*. Failure to integrate multiple input through the same sensory modality is termed an *intrasensory integrative disorder*. Intrasensory integrative dysfunctions involving the auditory system result in a form of auditory overloading. This leads to a breakdown in the organizational and selective processes of the system.

Luria (1966) states that the proper functioning of all higher mental systems requires the integrity of the entire brain, with all interconnections among the highly differential cortical areas working in harmony. He further states that circumscribed lesions in one area of the brain often manifest themselves in a group of disturbances involving several different systems.

Many studies have shown disturbances of intersensory systems in brain-damaged children. Birch and Belmont (1965) report a study in which these children exhibit greater problems in judgment using multisensory information than did normal children. In organizing their behavior, the brain-damaged children preferred to use more unisensory information (visual-visual). In another study, Belmont, Birch and Karp (1965) found that brain damage is associated with observable disturbances in both intersensory and intrasensory integration. They found, however, that the most marked disturbances occurred in intersensory integration. Birch and Lefford (1963) also found differences in the intersensory integrative ability between normal children and those with neurological impairment.

In a study of brain-damaged and normal adults, Benton et al. (1962) found that brain-damaged adults showed slower reaction times to stimuli that had been preceded by a different stimulus in the same sensory modality. Similar reaction times were found for both groups in changing from visual to auditory stimuli. When the auditory stimuli preceded visual stimuli the reaction time to the visual stimuli was significantly retarded in the brain-damaged adults. Among those adults with diffuse cerebral lesions more marked intersensory impairment was noted than among the normal controls and those with more focal lesions.

Thus, auditory perceptual problems might occur due to various defects: (1) problems in the temporal ordering (timing) of auditory impulses incident at the temporal cortex, (2) problems in the coding of auditory impulses at the terminal cortical areas of the temporal cortex, and (3) faulty transmission of impulses along the synaptic junctions of the brain stem. This system is the neurological alerting system which sensitizes certain cortical areas to respond to stimuli which are significant to them. This formation appears to have a filtering or *gating* function which also prevents noncritical stimuli from reaching prime cortical areas. Thus, the reticular formation is the attention-focusing system of the brain (Moruzzi and Magoun, 1949, Hebb, 1949, Bruner, 1958, and Desmedt, 1960). In this same vein, Mark (1969) mentions that there are often "additive losses" in children with minimal brain dysfunction where a malfunctioning system generates noise into other information-handling systems which might interfere with language comprehension during ordinary dialogue. This type of "additive loss" may well be due to a defect in the reticular formation.

Silver (1971) states that new knowledge in the disciplines of neurophysiology, neurochemistry and neuropharmacology make it possible to propose a view on the etiology of what he terms the "neurological learning disability syndrome." Specifically, he hypothesizes that this syndrome is the result of a neurohumoral deficiency resulting in physiological dysfunction of the ascending reticular formation and secondarily of the limbic system (see Fig. 6). Routtenberg (1968) postulated the existence of a second arousal system. This system is part of the limbic-midbrain system described anatomically by Nauta (1958). Upon stimulation with microelectrode implants, animals showed powerful reward (positive or negative) responses. This gives reason to assume that these areas are somehow basic to the neural mechanism of reward, incentive, motivation, affect, cognition and memory.

Both arousal systems are capable of causing neocortical desynchronization; however, the reticular formation appears to be more critical. The reticular formation dysfunction can be

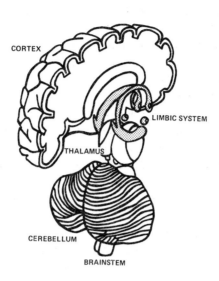

Figure 6. Anatomical location of the limbic system.

differentiated from the limbic system by way of the hippocampal theta activity; therefore, a positive feedback loop exists between the ascending reticular formation and the neocortex. Apparently at low or intermediate levels of activity the limbic system predominates over the reticular formation since the suppressing effect of hippocampal theta activity tends to diminish the positive-feedback effect between the reticular formation and the neocortex. At high levels of activity, however, the reticular formation predominates since the feedback system's activity will be too great to be suppressed by hippocampal theta activity.

In his work with cats, Grastyan (1959) found that in the relationship between the two arousal systems, the reticular formation predominates in the process of learning when exposed to new, novel, unfamiliar stimuli as well as during exposure to stimuli so familiar as to call forth automatic learned responses. Thus, he reasons that while the reticular formation is vital in terms of activating or alerting the organism to attend stimuli and to emit appropriate responses, it is the limbic system that predominates during the actual learning process.

Thus, the two arousal systems function in an integrated manner, each suppressing the activity of the other. This reciprocal inhibition allows for a state of dynamic equilibrium between the two systems, and an imbalance in one affects the functioning of the other.

While exploring the behavioral disturbances resulting when organisms are exposed to conditions of sensory distortion, deprivation or overload, Lindsley (1961) suggested that the role of the reticular formation is to act as a physiological barometer which adjusts or regulates input-output relations. Any conditions of sensory deprivation, overload or distortion upset the regulatory balance of the system with resulting disruption to perception and attention.

Thus, the reticular formation activates the neocortex so it can respond appropriately to incoming stimuli; it inhibits sensory input (gating and/or filtering function), thereby avoiding overloading the cortex; it also appears to facilitate motor output from the neocortex, thereby allowing for purposeful, organized muscle activity. Dysfunction of the reticular formation could result in (1) decreased inhibition of sensory input, resulting in cortical overloading; (2) decrease in the gating or selective arousal of the neocortex, resulting in poorer discrimination of sensory input; and (3) decrease in facilitation of neocortical motor output, resulting in an increase in apparent random or purposeless motor activity. Any alteration in the functioning of the limbic system would result in difficulties with perception, attention, learning, memory, drive, reward, motivation, incentive and affect.

Therefore, in considering the two arousal systems as a whole and their effects should dysfunction occur, Silver (1971) feels that a decreased functioning of the reticular formation could explain the clinical findings of hyperactivity, distractability and short attention span. The secondary dysfunction of the limbic system could explain the learning problems, perseveration, poor motivation and emotional lability associated with MBD.

The anatomy of the reticular formation, according to Minckler (1972), almost defies structural definition because of its ubiquity and scattering. It is not surprising, therefore, that this nonspecific, multisynaptic ascending and decending neuronal chain has been overshadowed in man by the more easily demonstrable principal neural pathways.

The fibers and cells of the spinal reticular system interlink with medullary reticular formation via the spinoreticular and reticulospinal tracts. This medullary portion of the system is called reticuloreticular. Neural input into the reticular formation includes multisynaptic and collateral chains from the spinal cord, cerebellum, hypothalamus, spinal and cranial nerves, the cerebral cortex, limbic system and basal nuclei.

Minckler describes the functions of the reticular formation in this manner:

> All known major pathways pour collaterals into the reticular formation. The system therefore represents an alternate means of conveying signals arising in the specific modalities from the principal paths to many relay stations and reflex systems. In general this system is regarded as a route by which a stimulus pattern can influence other neural activity rather than as an alternate pathway for conveying sensation to conscious centers .... Another function is that of alerting or preparatory activation (sometimes inhibition) of the neuronal pools, so that normal major pathway or integrative sequences can be carried out. Some degree of localization is apparent in the facilitory-inhibitory function. Experimental stimulation of the rostral part of the brainstem reticular formation (midbrain and thalamus) produces facilitation, while inhibition results from stimulation of the caudal part (medullary). It appears that the reticulospinal tract represents an important extrapyramidal motor pathway from basal nuclei to the final-common-path cells .... The reticular system thus enters into numerous emotional and behavorial responses in either suppressing or facilitating them. As a component of the alerting and arousal mechanism, the converse might be expected, and the system does play a role in sleep and coma.

The other arousal system, the limbic system, is described by Minckler (1972) as follows:

> The limbic system has adapted a combination of the neocortex and rhinencephalon to the efferent needs relating to *affect* to general sensibility. While structurally manifest in the

temporal lobe and hippocampal structures that discharge into hypothalamus via the fornices, the system is much more complex. The limbic outflow comingles in the thalamus with visceral influences arising from all sensory complexes as well as associative cortical areas, and culminates in behavioral responses. A strong relationship exists with autonomic and neuroendocrine functions, although a separation of these three systems (limbic, neuroendocrine, and autonomic) does to some degree occur in the thalamus and its output.

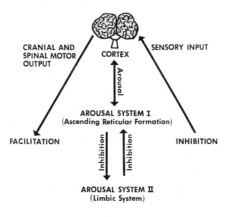

CRANIAL AND SPINAL MOTOR OUTPUT

CORTEX

SENSORY INPUT

Arousal

AROUSAL SYSTEM I (Ascending Reticular Formation)

FACILITATION

Inhibition   Inhibition

INHIBITION

AROUSAL SYSTEM II (Limbic System)

Figure 7. The relationship between the cortex and the reticular formation and the limbic arousal systems (after Silver, 1971).

See Figure 7 for the relationship between the cortex and the reticular formation and the limbic arousal systems.

THE LIMBIC SYSTEM: LEARNING AND MEMORY

Instantly available memory seems to be a function of the primary sensory cortex. Thus, patients having hippocampal lesions do not appear to have the required temporary storage for retaining readily available memory while attending other stimuli. So we see that the hippocampus serves in such cases rather as an intermediate storage for engrams representing stimuli in order to secure their retention. This preserves engrams from being disrupted in the primary memory storage of the sensory cortex itself. Immediate memory storage is necessary for tasks requiring sequential discrimination and for those memories whose importance has yet to be determined, and the relative value of whose place, if any, in memory storage is still to be assessed (Smythies, 1969 and 1970). Milton (1963) suggests that the hippocampus acts as a mechanism to protect memory traces during the critical stage of their consolidation. Douglas (1967), however, believes that the main function of the hippocampus is to enable an organism to balance responses with the stimulus received by the inhibition of a prepotent response. In his experiments with rats, Douglas was able to show that hippocampal lesions do not interfere with the rodents' ability to learn sequential responses as such so long as their successful execution does not involve the need to inhibit an established response to a stimulus.

A correlation of human data and results of animal experiments suggests, therefore, that an important function of the hippo-campus may be to store recent memory patterns and segments of behavioral patterns where both are free from disruption by dis-tracting influences, but nevertheless are instantly available to those mechanisms that actually organize ongoing behavior or permanent memory formation. The hippocampus could also have a more active function, i.e. "Integrating complex engrams which represent a sensory inflow integrating with related items called up from memory storage in a sort of template operation. In this way the input can be analyzed and categorized so in turn, the most appropriate S-R bonds can be effected." Another idea is that a peripheral mechanism may exert control over response-inhibition simply by inhibiting the organism's attention to the unwanted stimulus. This could be done either by the hippo-campus' function of reciprocally inhibiting the reticular forma-tion or by gating the sensory input at the geniculate level (Smythies, 1969).

The Limbic System and Neuroendocrine Control

Other well-established functions of the hippocampus are the tonic inhibition it exerts over the organism's pituitary adrenal stress mechanism and it's control over secretion of ovarian hormones. Thus, the hippocampus has important neuroendocrine properties and acts as a feedback control mechanism in opposition to the amygdala (Smythies, 1969, 1970).

The amygdala has important visceral connections and exerts a higher control of the hypothalamus, i.e. a push and pull force over such hypothalamic functions as eating and drinking. Lesions here delay the rise of plasma-free cortisone in the blood following immobilization stress. The amygdala appears to play a significant role in conditioning and learning. It also seems to play the important function of interrelating different reinforcement stimuli and modulating ongoing behavior. It also may have a mutually inhibitory relationship with the reticular formation in the process of arousal and attention (Smythies, 1969).

Delgado (1964) thinks that the limbic system is concerned with planning behavior and effecting its organization into a coherent sequence. It does this by linking together or activating preformed behavioral sequences whose engrams are stored in other areas such as the hypothalamus.

We may conclude that memory formation, conditioned reflexes, motivational patterns and many other higher mental functions are mediated largely by elements of the limbic system with the hippocampus and the amygdala playing a central role.

Consequently, in the normally functioning brain we can picture a memory and belief-generating system involving circuits based on the hippocampus and the reticular formation. This system is modulated in turn by circuits based on the amygdala and reticular formation which mediate variables in reinforcement and motivation. Smythies (1967 and 1969) feels that in this manner emotional reactions and beliefs are determined by the patterns formed by experiences. Because of some biochemical or cybernetic disturbance, however, the amygdala-based circuits may become dominant over those of the hippocampus. In this way the causal chain may reverse. If this reversal occurs, beliefs, even perceptions, would become determined by emotional factors.

The Limbic System and Schizophrenia

Smythies (1969) expands these ideas further to explain the

many bizarre symptoms of schizophrenia. One biochemical hypothesis of causation concerns the metabolism of noradrenalin and serotonin. Both of these appear to act as key neurotransmitters in the limbic system. Since its function is to coordinate perception, thinking, emotions and behavior, any extensive disruption of its biochemistry would lead also to a general breakdown in these vital functions:

> Such resulting symptoms as thought blockage, ideas of thought insertion or removal, a variety of perceptual distortions, or incongruity of affect, etc., lend themselves readily to explanations or a mechanical failure in the thinking process or in the mechanisms serving to correlate the various mental functions. In mechanisms whose smooth operation is normally taken for granted, the totally unfamiliar effect of these disorders on the subject may occasion secondary delusional effects as the subject tries to adjust to his disturbed condition. In later stages his disorder could involve the temporal lobe cortex as well. Generally, however, the intellectual functions in schizophrenia, which presumably depend mainly on the cholinergic mechanisms of the neocortex, are well preserved. Thus I would suggest that many so-called bizarre symptoms of schizophrenia can be accounted for if we regard the disease as a result of a disturbance in those biochemical mechanisms that are utilized in synaptic transmission in crucial areas of the limbic system including its important components in the temporal lobe.

To summarize, we can simply say that the hippocampus stores memories and with the amygdala determines what memories are to be retained. Subserving this process, the reticular formation provides the required complex switching and program organization needed for reception, evaluation, storage and instant recall. Thus, the entire limbic system functions to select and provide the appropriate behavior pattern for reacting effectively to any given set of stimuli received. In this context the cortex may be considered as a "specialized computing subsystem" to solve the problems of great complexity and in the process to supply the needed memory storage, social and spatial analyses, and language functions (Smythies, 1966 and 1970).

Chapter 4

DIAGNOSTIC CONSIDERATIONS

THE incidence of minimal brain dysfunction (MBD) among gradeschool children is not truly known. This fact reflects the chaotic state of our often-superficial diagnostic and remedial efforts in the field. Yet we must face the reality that the disorder does exist, and we must employ the tools we have at present to meet the problem. It is of little benefit to today's child with MBD to wait with us on future diagnostic and therapeutic procedures which will have been subjected to greater scientific evaluation.

Wunderlich (1968) reports the preliminary results of an incidence report by the National Institute of Neurological Disease and Blindness, which indicated that 14 percent of the entire child population had some degree of neurologic dysfunction by the end of the sixth year of life. Parnell and Korzeniowski (1972) state that auditory perceptual disturbances are found in 46 to 70 percent of children with learning disabilities.

Although the majority of these children have normal or above-average IQ's, they become underachievers due to their perceptual disabilities. It is extremely important that this type of child be recognized and diagnosed early so remedial steps may be taken to augment perceptual strengths and offset weaknesses. Table IV provides an auditory perceptual checklist for parents and teachers which should aid in early recognition of possible problems.

Lovitt (1967) advocates a behavioral method for the evaluation of children with learning disabilities based on a four-point assessment procedure: (1) baseline assessment, (2) assessment of behavioral components, (3) assessment based on referral, and (4) generalization of assessment.

The baseline assessment is a continual assessment of behavior until a stable, specified level of performance is reached. This ongoing diagnosis can then be compared to the more indirect measures such as standardized test scores.

The assessment of behavioral components is the evaluation of

58

TABLE IV

AUDITORY PERCEPTUAL CHECK LIST

Name _____Sex _____ Date _____

	Yes	No
1. Is generally aware of sounds objects make	___	___
Is generally aware of sounds animals make	___	___
2. Can associate sound with object	___	___
Can associate object with sound	___	___
3. Has difficulty remembering names, dates, times, places, rhythmic patterns (specify).................................	___	___
4. Is easily distracted by extraneous noises	___	___
5. Appears to cock one ear toward the teacher or other sources of sound	___	___
6. Shows excessive reaction to loud sounds......................	___	___
7. Appears to have a speech problem	___	___
8. Poor memory span for numbers, sounds, connected speech, directions, and so on	___	___
9. Inability to discriminate between similar sounding words	___	___
10. Can repeat sounds, letters, syllables, words, phrases, sentences, numbers and main events of stories in proper sequence	___	___
11. Has difficulty interpreting meaning of words, phrases, sentences or stories...	___	___
12. Frequently asks for things to be repeated	___	___
13. Has difficulty spelling words that are dictated to him...........	___	___
14. Appears to focus on only part of what is said	___	___
15. Leaves out a number of words when asked to repeat words or sentences..	___	___
16. Has difficulty locating the source of sounds not in line of vision..	___	___

REMARKS:

_____
_____
_____

Observer_____ Specialist_____

those behavioral components that maintain and modify a child's behavior. For example, (1) the type and quality of the stimulus materials presented to the child and the degree of choice he is allowed to exercise in selecting his stimulus materials and the rate at which they are presented to him, (2) the contingency requirements of the child or how many consequences are necessary to affect performance, (3) the number and effect of the child's responses in his continuously changing environment; and (4) the environmental consequencies that maintain behavior. Many times direct observation of how the child interacts and reacts to stimuli in his environment is necessary.

The assessment based on referral involves the parents and teachers in the evaluation process. The competency of the home and school situations to deal with the child's perceptual problem must be assessed. Also, the goals of the referring party must be taken into account in planning any remedial program.

Following the *generalization of assessment*, the diagnostic information provided for the teachers and parents should result in immediate program implementation for the child. All processes and tests employed during the diagnosis should be clearly stated.

GENERAL DIAGNOSTIC SIGNS*

The general diagnostic signs of minimal brain dysfunction include the following:

1. Hyperkinesis is characterized by the child's hyperactive, restless, disruptive, disorganized and impulsive behavior.

2. Hypokinesis is characterized by the child's slowness in movement, thinking and talking.

3. Distractibility is evident as the child is unable to ignore ambient noises, inconsequential movement and stimuli. This poor concentration often manifests itself in a short attention span.

4. Low emotional threshold leads to emotional overreaction to situations; the child cries and laughs inappropriately and sometimes displays undue aggression.

5. Abnormal speech development includes such problems as delayed speech and language, poor articulation and echolalia (inappropriate repetition of what someone else has said).

6. Poor motor coordination is often displayed in the child's awkwardness in running and skipping and in his ungainly or clumsy gait. A low diadochokinetic rate, or the inability to perform rapid alternating movements, can be observed in the child's poor skipping ability, especially in changing leads, and in his inability to perform rapid tongue and lip movements.

---

*Modified from Clements (1966).

7. Perseveration is characterized by excessive repetition of a specific behavior or language pattern after it ceases to be functional.

Other equivocal neurological signs sometimes noted are transient strabismus, mixed and/or confused laterality, poor hand-eye coordination, electroencephalographic irregularities and a high incidence of allergies. It is most important that these signs not be used in making haphazard nonclinical or *guess* diagnoses of minimal brain dysfunction. Such diagnoses should only be made by qualified professionals after all the medical, social, psychological and educational information is taken into consideration.

Prentky (1972) concludes that despite the multiplicity of symptoms in MBD, certain symptoms do tend to cluster into recognizable clinical entities. He further suggests that these specific complexes of symptoms are subcategories within the general category of MBD.

Zach and Kaufman (1972) caution educators not to apply indiscriminate designations to children as perceptually handicapped. They grant that some children have perceptual problems which interfer with their success in school. They question, however, the ability to identify these problems, define these problems and train such children to become successful learners. The critical task for educators is to delineate how children perceive, what they perceive and through what sensory channels they process information. In order to truly understand the perceptual process, one must consider it developmentally with developmental norms established at each age level.

Denhoff et al. (1972) found that major and minor neurologic signs observable at birth and in the first year are clearly associated with inefficient learning skills and poor school performance at age seven. Their observations of 380 children over a seven-year period lead to the development of Stress Indexes compiled during the first year of birth. These include

1. Birth Stress Index — Stress items from the obstetric record and from a newborn diagnostic summary.

2. First Year Stress Index — Birth stress items were combined with stress items from the pediatric summary of the first year.

3. Neonatal Outcome Index — Was made up of outcome (observable signs of inadequate neurodevelopment in the child) items from the newborn diagnostic summary.

4. First Year Outcome Index — Was made up of neonatal outcome index and outcome items from the summary of the first year.

These observations promote the possibility of developing an index which may be useful in helping to identify the baby who is at risk for later development of learning problems. The authors caution that their results are preliminary at this time and that their Outcome Index is not yet ready for clinical trial. They point out that until an objective rating scale is ready, the greatest number of their suspicious cases stemmed from the *hypoactive* and *hyperreactive* categories, with other minor diagnostic signs such as lethargy, abnormal cry, jitteriness, or tremulousness, and hyperactive behavior being the most frequent.

The authors point to the need for further refinement of their Outcome Index, to the need for parent education for those parents with *difficult-to-mother* babies, and for early identification and long-term follow-up of various social classes of high risk babies and their normal controls. This is perhaps the only way to resolve the inherent uncertainties in the concept of minimal brain dysfunction and possibly discover a neurologic basis for those cases with adverse outcome in later life. The real worth of environmental enrichment programs can be explored in a similar manner.

It is of interest to note that Rosenblith (1961), using a modified Graham Behavior Test for Neonates with the Denhoff sample, has been able to identify a small sample of light-sensitive babies who later turned out to be neurologically impaired. He found also that a discrepancy in muscle tension between extremities, with upper limb flaccidity and lower limb hypertonicity, is an unfavorable prognostic sign.

In his discussion of the physical findings upon ENT (ear, nose and throat) examination of children with suspected MBD, Merifield (1970) explains that the physical examination is often difficult and that this difficulty itself should be a clue to the diagnosis. The child must often touch every object in sight, and frequently asks what is this and that. He squirms and grimaces and cannot sit still. Often he will cooperate for a period, then suddenly become stubborn or cry and cling to his mother. In addition to the routine ENT examination, Merifield performs a brief neurological examination:

1. Motility-Posture Tests — A normal three-year-old can stand on one foot momentarily. A six-year-old should be adept at this. Normal four to five-year-olds can walk a straight line and have no trouble with left-to-right turns.

2. Fine Motor Coordination — Finger-to-thumb opposition should be performed easily by a four-year-old. Brain-damaged children have difficulty with the release phenomenon and with touching the fingers in sequence. They may skip fingers in the attempt. The handicapped child is often unable to hold his hands extended while concentrating on another task. Extrapyramidal involvement is often seen in this task as drifting of the hands with convergence and divergence. A spreading of the fingers with hands extended may be a sign of cerebellar disease.

TESTS FOR AUDITORY PERCEPTUAL PROBLEMS

The basic audiological battery should always be performed first. It is necessary that testing other than air conduction pure-tone screening be performed in a sound-treated booth by an audiologist who holds the Certificate of Clinical Competence from the American Speech and Hearing Association or any equivalent foreign certification. In 1954, Myklebust pointed to an expanded role for the audiologist in the area of receptive disorders in children with these words:

> Currently the audiologist is oriented more to the problems of impaired auditory acuity and to adults than to the auditory disorders of infants and young children. However, interest and research in the area of young children is developing rapidly. As this work develops the audiologist will find it necessary to be more comprehensive and to become oriented to receptive language disorders in general. In terms of differential diagnosis of children, this entails a background in such problems as receptive aphasia and psychic deafness in children. The audiologist

can be expected to devise differential tests of auditory acuity and tests for other types of auditory disorders.

The basic battery consists of pure-tone air and bone conduction tests, speech reception threshold (SRT) and speech discrimination tests using phonetically-balanced (PB) word lists. Phonetically-balanced kindergarten word lists may be used with children under six years; and for children without expressive language, word intelligibility tests based on picture identification are usually employed. Advanced tests for differential diagnosis are generally not employed by the audiologist unless a conductive (middle ear) or sensorineural (cochlear) pathology exists.

In his attempt to devise a developmental test of auditory perception, Abramovitz (1971) points to the ephemeral nature of sound itself as a prime reason for the lack of items on intelligence tests for children that are directly concerned with the basic skills related to auditory perception. In a physical sense, complex sound can be analyzed along three basic parameters — frequency, intensity and time. A naturalistic psychological classification should include (a) the perception and integration of the ambient auditory environment (natural, mechanical and other sounds), (b) the perception of tones and organized acoustic patterns, and (c) the perception of speech sounds. Abramovitz (1971) states that a viable clinical test of auditory perception would have to meet the following criteria:

1. The "floor" of the test had to be low enough to establish the level of the youngest, most handicapped child who was capable of being subjected to a rigorous testing procedure (though ostensibly presented as a "game").

2. The "ceiling" of the test had to be high enough to establish the level of the most well-endowed primary school child.

3. The method of administration was to be such that children with communication handicaps would not be at a disadvantage in comparison with children not so handicapped.

4. As far as possible, only the auditory modality was to be under scrutiny, which meant trying to exclude cross-modality and coordination functions, e.g. audiovisual and audiomotor skills as such.

5. Administration of the test should not take more than half

an hour. Alternatively, each section should not take longer than fifteen minutes.

6. The reliabilities and Standard Errors of Measurement of each subtest should be such as to produce an effective instrument for individual assessment.

Since Abramovitz (1971) recognized the need for such a qualitative and quantitative psychological assessment of the child's auditory abilities and disabilities, he devised a test designed to evaluate the following functions: (a) recognition of environmental sounds, (b) auditory figure-ground discrimination, (c) speech-sound discrimination (phonemic and intonational), and (d) tonal pattern discrimination (pitch, loudness, duration and interval). The test was given to 205 children, ages five to ten years, drawn from a normal school population, and 232 children with difficulties and handicaps of varying degree and kind.

Only the first two subtests were found to be both clinically and experimentally viable. Brain-injured, retarded, emotionally disturbed and *normal* children with average intelligence with reading and/or spelling difficulties generally test low on auditory figure-ground discrimination. As discussed earlier in Chapter 3, difficulty in discriminating the figure from the ground may be due to reticular formation and limbic system dysfunction.

The standardized tests of auditory perception may be given by trained professionals other than audiologists. Specialized testing techniques of discrimination ability employing a high signal-to-noise ratio and/or high- and low-pass filter units, as well as sound-field localization tasks and localization tests under earphones should be performed by the audiologist in that a controlled sound environment is needed requiring the use of sophisticated audiometric equipment and techniques.

Tests of auditory perception consist of The Wepman Discrimination Test (1958), the auditory sections of the Illinois Test of Psycholinguistic Abilities (Kirk, McCarthy, and Kirk, 1968), the Auditory Analysis Test (Rosner and Simon, 1970), the Screening Test of Auditory Perception (Kimmell and Wahl, 1969), the Auditory-Visual Pattern Test (Birch and Belmont, 1965), the auditory sections of the Rosner Perceptual Survey (1969), The Roswell-Chall Auditory Blending Test (1963), The Lindamood

Auditory Conceptualization Test (1971), and the memory span tests adapted from the Stanford-Binet and Wechsler scales.

The *Wepman Discrimination Test* examines the child's ability to recognize single-feature differences, for example sounds differing in only a single phoneme. The child listens to two words, e.g. sick-thick, bead-deed, and tells whether the two words sound alike or different. False-choice items, e.g. chew-chew, in which the words are truly alike are intermingled with the test items. Normal five-year-old children will make less than seven errors; seven-year-olds, less than five errors; and eight-year-olds, less than four errors. Over the age of eight no more than three errors can be considered within normal range. The child is expected to have the concepts of like and different. Wepman (1960) has shown a high correlation between failure on this test and the prediction of reading difficulties, especially in regard to phonics.

The auditory decoding, auditory-vocal association, auditory closure, sound blending, and auditory sequential memory subtests to the Illinois Test of Psycholinguistic Abilities (ITPA) are often employed in auditory perceptual testing along with those subtests which measure visual and motor areas.

Auditory Reception (Decoding). With this test the child's ability to understand verbally presented material is assessed. The child is required to give a yes or no response to fifty such questions as, "Do ants crawl?" "Do clowns tumble?" "Do leaves flutter?" The test items are given until the child fails three items in any of seven items consecutively presented. The vocabulary in successive items becomes increasingly difficult while the expected responses remain at the two-year age level.

Auditory-Vocal Association. The child's ability to manipulate linguistic symbols in a meaningful way is tested by his completing forty-two analogous sentences presented such as "A bird flies in the air; a fish swims in the ____"; "On my hands I have fingers; on my feet I have ____."

Auditory Closure. This test assesses the child's ability to fill in the parts of words deleted in an auditory presentation and to speak the words thus completed. The child is presented thirty items of increasing difficulty, for example airpla/ and / ype / iter.

Sound Blending. Sounds composing a word are spoken singly at half-second intervals, and the child must combine the sounds so as to tell what the word is. In Section A of the test, words are divided into two to three sounds each and presented with picture cues such as, "Listen. F-OOT. Which one am I talking about?" In Section B, words are presented as before but without picture cues, and the words are divided into two to seven sounds each. In Section C, nonsense words of three to six sounds each with diacritical markings to distinguish long and short vowel sounds are presented, for example "What is this? Z-E."

Auditory Sequential Memory. In this test the child's ability to reproduce digital sequences increasing in length from two to eight digits is tested. This test differs from the digital memory tasks of the Stanford-Binet and the Wechsler Intelligence Scales for Children in that the representation rate for the digits is two per second and that the child is given a second trial at each sequence if he fails to reproduce the initial presentation.

The *Auditory Analysis Test* (AAT) consists of forty words varying in length from one to four syllables. The testee is requested to repeat a spoken word, then to repeat it again without certain specified phonemic elements, e.g. a beginning, ending or medially-positioned consonant sound. Seven categories of item difficulty are given. The authors were seeking a measure of phonic analysis and synthesis behavior which requires encoding responses more complex than the usual yes-no discriminations. With this test the child is asked to remember and analyze spoken sounds and to demonstrate these abilities in his oral responses. The test can be administered to kindergarten through grade six children.

The *Screening Test for Auditory Perception* (STAP) is a group screening test consisting of five parts for grades two through six. The subtests measure the child's ability to recognize the two basic vowel sounds — long and short — when contained in words, the child's ability to differentiate between initial single consonant sounds and blends, ability to discriminate between rhyming and nonrhyming words, the child's ability to retain and identify sound patterns, and the child's ability to detect subtle differences in paired words.

The *Auditory-Visual Pattern Test* was developed to test the relationship between a temporarily-structured set of auditory stimuli and a spatially-distributed set of visual stimuli. The examiner taps out patterns (tap-tap-tap). The testee is then shown three visual patterns (...) (..) (.) and is instructed to "pick out the dots which look like the taps you hear." This test was found to be a successful predictor in differentiating children with lower and higher reading scores.

The auditory sections of the *Rosner Perceptual Survey* (RPS) consist of a word repetition and an auditory organization task as well as the Birch and Belmont Auditory-Visual Pattern Test already discussed.

Roswell-Chall Auditory Blending Test. This evaluates a child's ability to combine and blend sounds to form words when the sounds are presented orally. Since the test is given orally, the child does not have to be able to associate the sounds with the corresponding letters or to syllabify words heard. The test may be given to children grades one through four and to older children who exhibit reading difficulties. The sounds are given at a rate of about one-half second for each sound and only one trial is given for each word. The child is instructed to blend the sounds as spoken by the examiner and say the word they form, e.g. c-ow, t-ime, m-a-p. Children with adequate blending score as follows:

Grade 1	7 of 30 test items
Grade 2	11 of 30 test items
Grade 3	15 of 30 test items
Grade 4	19 of 30 test items
Grade 5 or above	26 of 30 test items

Children who score below these scores are said to have inferior auditory blending skills or inability to break down components of words.

The *Lindamood Auditory Conceptualization Test* (LAC Test) indicates the child's level of auditory functioning along two indices: (1) the child's ability to discriminate one speech sound from another — same or different — and (2) the child's ability to perceive the number and order of sounds in sequences, both in nonsyllabic and syllabic patterns. The child is required to manipulate colored wooden blocks to arbitrarily represent sounds given by the tester. No consistent relationship exists between specific colors and specific sounds other than to denote the repetition of the same sound within a pattern or a set of patterns. The test is given in two segments. In the first segment the child is required to discriminate how many sounds he heard, their sameness or difference, and the order he heard them. In the second segment the child represents changes in syllabic patterns as a sound is added, substituted, omitted, shifted or repeated by moving the colored blocks from a basic pattern to show the changes in sounds or order of the pattern. Nonsense syllables can be substituted as needed to eliminate the possibility of responses being influenced by familiarity with meaningful words. The authors contend that this test can be used with students of all ages, presumably from first grade on.

Often the Gray's Oral Reading Paragraphs (1955) are used as a measure of sight-reading ability due to their simplicity of administration and content of the paragraphs. A formal scoring sheet is provided, and the child is asked to read aloud beginning with a paragraph two grade levels below his present grade placement. Care should be taken to ascertain the time of the school year when determining reading level. The number and type of errors are recorded while the child reads along with speed, smoothness, approach (phonetic, or not) and comprehension of the material.

A useful tool in quickly obtaining an impression of the child's overall capacity to gain and use language as a tool is the *Communicative Evaluation Chart From Infancy to Five Years* (Anderson, Miles and Matheny, 1963). The items evaluated indicate whether or not the child should be referred for further evaluation.

The basic study of short-term memory is to assess the stimulus afterimage. The afterimage arises from the excitation of neurons after a stimulus is presented. Assessment based on the duration of the afterimage's direct retention affects the essential processes of the memory function.

Memory Span

Widely-used measures of auditory memory span involve the use of digits, words, sentences, nonsense syllables, paragraphs and stories which are to be recalled following a single presentation. When the number of stimuli presented is increased, the examiner is able to test the number of elements the subject is able to retain and retrieve. Some variables that affect retention are (1) nature and quantity of previously-acquired information, (2) what remains to be learned, (3) extent of practice received, (4) the rate at which the items are presented, (5) amount of practice given, (6) the familiarity and significance of the material to the subject, (7) how well the subject can reinterpret and articulate it, (8) the subject's energy level at the time of day of the presentation, (9) the distractions present during presentation, (10) methods used in test scoring, and (11) the subject's psychological and physiological states at the time (Lumley and Calhoun, 1934, and Underwood, 1964).

Delayed Memory Response

Tests of delayed memory response require call backs and responses to dormant stimuli. The child must recall what or where the stimulus was. Two questions in delayed response testing are (1) how long can a symbol be retained to facilitate recall and (2) how many of the items presented can be retrieved. The interval between presentation and recall can be lengthened until the child fails to recall the text items (Hunter, 1957).

Procedures for evaluating memory, both for the short and long-term are greatly needed. These should give weight to the quality and meaningfulness of the material, the learning steps needed for retention, anticipated duration of the retention period, and extraneous stimuli and activities introduced during the expected retention period. Perhaps we should evaluate memory more in terms of specific school tasks requiring recall and recognition for successful task completion.

AN ABBREVIATED DIAGNOSTIC BATTERY

In order to test the diagnostic significance of an abbreviated test battery for children with auditory perceptual problems due to minimal brain dysfunction, this author tested thirty children with learning problems and thirty normal children as a control group. Four standardized tests were given: The Wepman Test of Auditory Discrimination, the Rosner Auditory Analysis Test, the Roswell-Chall Auditory Blending Test, and the Binet Sentence Memory Test. See this chapter for an explanation of these tests.

Method

Thirty children with learning problems were divided into three groups according to age (6, 7 and 8 years), with ten children in each age group. All children had normal acuity for hearing by routine air, bone and speech audiometry. Each child in the experimental group had average to above-average intelligence but all attended one or two private schools for children with learning disabilities.

All experimental children exhibited the diagnostic signs of reading problems, poor attention span (distractability) and hyperkinetic activity. Males outnumbered females two to one in the experimental group (20 males and 10 females). Thirty normal children also ages six through eight years (18 males and 12 females) served as a control group.

Each child was seated in a sound-treated room during testing. While being tested, the children were in an *auditory isolated* situation in that they could not see the tester who was seated behind a one-way mirror in the test suite. Preliminary test instructions were given to the child face-to-face prior to testing. Test items were given over a speech microphone incorporated into a Maico MA-10 audiometer and were received by the child through stereophonic speakers at either side, eight feet apart. The test data was collected between February 1972 and September 1973.

Results

The following table shows the results of the statistical treatment of the data. Mean, variance, standard deviations and statistical comparisons for the experimental and the control groups on the four standardized tests are shown. The t values were significant at the 0.01 level of confidence for all the tests except for the

Auditory Perceptual Disorders

Binet Sentence Memory Test for the seven and eight-year-old children; however t values were significant at the 0.05 level of confidence for these age group.

TABLE V

DATA FOR MEAN, VARIANCE, STANDARD
DEVIATIONS AND STATISTICAL COMPARISONS
FOR THE EXPERIMENTAL AND CONTROL
GROUPS ON FOUR STANDARDIZED TESTS

Test	Experimental Group (N=30)			Control Group (N=30)			Difference		
Auditory Analysis	Mean	Variance	SD	Mean	Variance	SD	Means	Diff. of SD	*t
6 yrs.	3.7	5.122	2.263	17.8	11.288	3.359	14.1	1.281	11.007
7 yrs.	6.3	12.455	3.529	21.4	21.155	4.599	15.1	1.833	8.236
8 yrs.	9.7	16.233	4.029	26.2	21.733	4.666	16.5	1.948	8.468
Roswell-Chall									
6 yrs.	2.3	3.788	1.946	10.0	2.888	1.699	7.7	.817	9.423
7 yrs.	5.0	7.555	2.748	16.6	11.822	3.438	11.6	1.392	8.333
8 yrs.	9.1	10.100	3.178	24.5	17.388	4.170	15.4	1.657	9.288
Wepman									
6 yrs.	10.6	5.822	2.412	2.1	1.877	1.370	8.5	.877	9.687
7 yrs.	7.8	4.622	2.149	.7	.455	.674	7.1	.712	9.963
8 yrs.	6.2	3.733	1.932	.6	.711	.843	5.6	.666	8.400
Sentence Memory									
6 yrs.	5.8	2.400	1.549	7.5	.277	.527	1.7	.517	3.285
7 yrs.	6.7	1.566	1.251	7.7	.156	.395	1.0	.415	2.409
8 yrs.	8.7	2.677	1.636	10.5	3.611	1.900	1.8	.793	2.269

*With 18 degrees of freedom (df), a t value of 2.878 at the 0.01 level of confidence is significant; a t value of 2.101 at the 0.05 level of confidence is significant.

Discussion

No overlapping of the test scores between the two groups was seen except on the Binet Sentence Memory Test at the seven and eight-year levels. Although the scoring criterion is rather strict on this test (errors include omissions, substitutions, additions, changes in words or in the order of words but not contractions), it did not differentiate the groups as clearly as the other three tests.

Errors were mostly common omissions, simplifications of items and ungrammatical repetitions. It appears that syntactical complexity rather than auditory memory per se is the critical factor in correct sentence repetition. The teaching of appropriate use of transformational structures and grammatical rules for future sentence regeneration appears to be indicated rather than rote memory exercises.

Obvious limitations exist in the use of standardized test scores. They cannot give a complete picture of the learning disabled child as to etiology, prognosis, psychological ramifications, nor indicate the optimum course for rehabilitation. Standardized test scores should, however, tell us quickly the areas of greatest weakness so a program of diagnostic teaching can be instituted. See Chapter 6 for a discussion of diagnostic teaching.

Among professionals in learning disorders there is a continual search for definitive tests which can be given quickly so as not to fatigue the child. The abbreviated diagnostic battery under discussion has the following advantages: (1) No more than twenty to thirty minutes are necessary to give all four tests and score them, allowing suspicions of auditory perceptual problems to be quickly confirmed. (2) Areas of greatest weakness in auditory perception (discrimination, blending and memory span) as they relate to the major signs of learning disabilities associated with MBD can be quickly ascertained for more in-depth study as a program of diagnostic teaching is instituted relative to the needs of the individual child.

Summary

The results of this study have shown that statistically-significant differences exist between the children with learning problems and the normal control group for the four standardized tests. The results therefore indicate that these differences can be applied to the differential diagnosis of auditory perceptual disorders. By application of both the four standardized tests used in this study and the case history information relative to symptomatology and the learning problems involved, an additional diagnostic method is advanced to differentiate between normal children and children with auditory perceptual disorders (Barr, 1974).

Interdisciplinary Communication

Speech, voice and articulation testing as well as tests for language development are usually performed by certified speech and language pathologists. A team approach to the diagnosis and remediation of perceptual handicaps cannot be overemphasized. The professional disciplines of medicine, speech and language pathology, psychology, audiology, optometry, social work, and physical and occupational therapy supplement the work of the classroom teacher. The teacher acts as coordinator of the diagnostic and therapeutic information for classroom implementation. Problems in interdisciplinary communication often center around jurisdiction in decision-making situations, terminology, referral strategies and reporting practices in diagnosis and therapy (Bateman and Schiefelbusch, 1969). Continuing efforts at clarification of goals and improved communication and working relationships are essential (Clements, 1966).

THE ELECTROENCEPHALOGRAM (EEG) AND THE DIAGNOSIS OF MBD

Auditory information is conveyed from the inner ear to the brain by action potentials which travel along axons. The terminus of each axon makes contact with other nerve cells (neurons) in the brain at junctions called synapes. When the stimulus reaches a synapse, an ammonium compound, acetylcholine, is produced, causing the receptor fibers of the adjoining cell to be stimulated. An enzyme, cholinesterase, is instantly produced which destroys the acetylcholine (ACTH), leaving the nerve cells clear to receive further stimuli. This entire process takes approximately 4/10,000th of a second. It must be pointed out that the transmitter substance, ACTH, flowing across the synaptic cleft onto the outer membrane of the next cell (the postsynaptic cell) can be either excitatory or inhibitory — that is, it can either increase or decrease the probability that the postsynaptic cell will generate an action potential.

Information from each sensory end organ is processed along a separate sensory pathway. A sensory pathway consists of peripheral sense organs and several clusters of nerve cells called nuclei. Sensory information is processed in several stages so that each nucleus receives input from the preceding, processes the input, and sends the amplified and, in some cases, modified output on to the next nucleus. Each primary sensory pathway ends in a specific area of the cerebral cortex termed a *primary sensory receiving area.*

There are approximately thirteen billion neurons in the brain that constitute the fundamental cellular units of the nervous system. These nerve cells composed of body, dendrites and axon branches, function simultaneously in relay fashion as integrators and creators of electrical activity.

The EEG has, unfortunately, been touted by many in recent years as the last word in the diagnosis of minimal brain dysfunction and other neurological disorders. This is due in large measure to a misunderstanding of the diagnostic value and the limitations of the EEG. The diagnosis of MBD results from a summary of the test findings of all professional disciplines involved and not from test results of a single neurologic procedure.

Berger (1929) first published the results of his EEG recordings from human brains. Since that time, researchers have attempted to relate the EEG recordings of brain activity to behavioral experiences. One method of studying this relationship is to examine brain activity in response to presentations of closely-controlled stimulus inputs such as light flashes, sounds and tactile stimuli. These electrical potentials recorded from the brain are commonly called cortical evoked responses, and since these measured electrophysiologic changes in brain activity are beyond the voluntary control of the subject, the EEG is termed an objective measure (McCandless, 1971).

Figure 8 shows a schematic block diagram of an EEG setup featuring instrumentation used in stimulus presentation and data recording. All instruments are self-explanatory with the

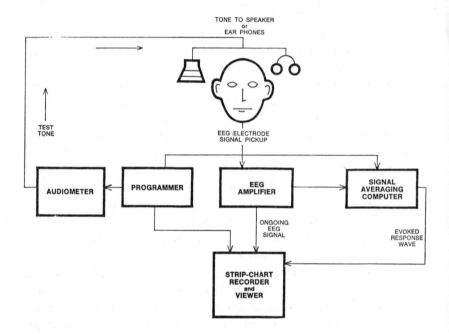

Figure 8. Electroencephalogram (EEG) block diagram for cortically evoked responses to sound stimuli.

exception of the computer. The computer is composed of a certain number of bins or channels (the number of bins varies according to the model of computer used). Each bin is assigned a certain segment of time, e.g. if one minute of activity is to be analyzed by a computer composed of thirty bins, each bin would be responsible for a designated two seconds of time. The electrical activity occurring during each segment of time is stored in its respective bin. Electrical activity which is unrelated to the stimuli will be cancelled out. After the computer has averaged or summed a predetermined number of stimuli, the voltage from each bin is displayed visually either on an oscilloscope or recorded on a graphic recorder.

Davis (1939) first described cortically-evoked responses in the human in response to auditory, visual and tactile stimuli. He called this response the "K Complex." At first this response was evoked from an area near the vertex of the head and was later called the "V Potential" (Bancaud, Bloch and Paippard, 1953). Now it is known that this response is diffused and can be measured at many areas of the head. The wave form is similar in pattern for all forms of stimulation, but minor latency and wave form differences exist for specific modalities. Taylor (1968) describes two components of the K complex — the slow delta wave and the fast activity, either of which may appear alone, with the fast activity more conspicuous in the central region and the slow delta more conspicuous in the frontal region. McCandless (1971) points out that the central pathways and structures which mediate a response to auditory stimuli are not known. Because of the long latencies associated with this response, associative structures in addition to the primary auditory areas of the temporal lobe may mediate the response. Frequency and voltage of oscillating potentials vary with the area of the brain recorded, the age and the state of consciousness of the subject.

The parameters which allow brain wave activity to be classified are the frequency (Hz), amplitude (in mv or microvolts), and the morphological and temporospatial characteristics. The four major wave forms are

1. The alpha ranges from 8 to 13 Hz and 30 to 50 mv in amplitude. This wave predominates in the posterior receptive fields and shows a typical spindle form. Its psychological correlates are restful wakefulness and relaxation. A blocking effect on this wave can occur with the performance of a single mental task or by opening the eyes. Waves in the same frequency range but measured from a more anterior location are called kappa waves; these are correlated with mental tasks and can persist with the eyes open.

2. Beta waves predominate in the anterior effective fields with a frequency of 14 to 26 Hz and an amplitude of 5 to 10 mv. These waves correlate with brain activation resulting from concentration and effort, and disappear during sleep. Faster brain waves exist up to several hundred cycles per second, but these have been little explored. Grastyan (1961) suggests that amygdala fast rhythm of 40 to 45 Hz (baso-lateral amygdala) indicates the general level of unconditioned mechanisms and drives and may also represent an alerting call to the amygdala for quick operation in conditions where its functions in reinforcement and reaction to meaningful stimuli and its role in alerting the pituitary-adrenal

axis may be called for.

3. Theta waves have a frequency of 4 to 7 Hz and are correlated with stages of light sleep, with children under thirteen years, and during exposure to new and novel situations. See Sklar et al. (1972) under "Cerebral Dominance and Auditory Perception" in Chapter 2. Adey (1967) feels that the hippocampal theta rhythm is not only associated with the orienting response (4-cycle rhythmicity) but has confirmed the presence of the six-cycle per second activity as a concomitant of discriminative behavior. The hippocampal theta rhythm is positively correlated with approach behavior, with the execution of a planned motor act, and with imprinting information of importance during the learning process. Its negative function is associated with rhythmic changes (desynchronization) which is the hippocampus' first response to novel stimuli and to the subsequent inhibition of the orienting response which is controlled by the reticular formation. Thereafter, if approach activity follows the orienting response, the hippocampus returns to action.

4. Delta waves have a frequency of 0.5 to 3.5 Hz and a large amplitude of 100 mv. This wave is typical of deep sleep and can be seen during infancy and in brain injury.

Banquet (1972, 1973) reported increased synchronization of waves in both cerebral hemispheres of subjects while meditating. These waves were characterized by a brief shift sequence of Alpha, Theta, Delta and a return to Alpha. The Alpha waves of 10 to 12 Hz were spread synchronously from the back to the front of the brain, implying possible increased integration of separate functions. Some indications, based on spectral analysis of the brain waves of these mediators, suggest a possible fourth state of consciousness achieved during meditation. Much remains to be investigated concerning the physiological changes which occur during meditation and during the use of biofeedback techniques and their relationship to perception and learning.

There appears to be no specific EEG abnormality associated with minimal brain dysfunction (Caputo, Niedermeyer, and Richardson, 1968). Hughes (1968) found the relationships between EEG abnormalities and test results of psychological functions in a population of learning disorders only when multivariant techniques were utilized with the aid of computer analysis.

It should not be concluded, however, that the EEG has no place in the diagnostic evaluation of patients suggesting minimal brain dysfunction. Indications for including an EEG recording are as follows: (1) sudden (paroxysmal) behavior abnormalities, (2) any history of obvious types of seizures (such as *petit mal* seizures), (3) a history of seizure equivalent behavior, and (4) a history suggesting progressive focal or global CNS dysfunction.

TESTS FOR CENTRAL AUDITORY LESIONS

One of the earliest and most comprehensive studies of the effects of speech and white noise on patients with temporal lobe lesions was done by Sinha (1959). In this study thirty-five patients with temporal lobe lesions, thirteen with lesions affecting cortical areas other than the temporal lobe and ten normal hearing subjects were tested. The test procedure included pure tone audiometry, speech reception thresholds, and speech discrimination testing (PB Max) without noise and with white noise. The PB words were presented at 35 dB (SL) in the presence of white noise at successively increasing levels (5 dB increments) from 10 to 35 dB.

Poorest scores on the discrimination test were found at white noise intensities of 25 to 30 dB for the contralateral ear, even when both ears were nearly equal for speech discrimination ability in the absence of noise. No marked superiority of the left as compared to the right temporal lobe was noted with regard to the auditory capacity tested. This finding could possibly be explained by the nature of the auditory stimuli presented which did not prove truly dichotic enough to elicit marked hemispheric dominance for verbal material.

Discrimination scores were worse prior to excision of the tumors. This could well be due to the foci of the tumor interfering with the neural-electrical activity of the brain which became less of a factor after the tumor was excised.

Jerger et al. (1968) sought to overcome some disadvantages in the traditional methodology of speech audiometry. The presentation of single-syllable phonetically-balanced (PB) words does not take into account the crucial parameter of the changing pattern of speech over time. In order to add this missing dimension it was necessary to develop materials based on relatively longer samples of speech than single words. Two other disadvantages of the traditional testing paradigm are the open message set and the problem of scoring the responses elicited. The open-set method does not control the subject's previous linguistic history and the extent to which this variable may affect his responses. A closed-set paradigm is preferable in that all possible responses to a given test item are rigidly specified.

The new speech materials developed are *synthetic*, synthetic in the sense that the sequence of words that comprise the sentences follow specifiable rules of syntax. Real sentences are not used because the meaning of such a sentence is often conveyed by only one or two key words. Most of the test sentences have seven words and nine syllables. The sequence of words in each successive sentence is a closer approximation to the kind of sequence one would normally expect to find with real English sentences. However, no word in the sentence is dependent on the word that precedes it. This, obviously, is unlike the natural events in language. See Appendix 2 for ten synthetic sentences.

In the testing procedure, unlike the traditional method, the patient identifies the message instead of repeating aloud what he hears. After each sentence presentation the patient searches a visually-presented list and tells the tester the number of the sentence he hears. The SSI procedure is presented via tape through a dual-channel audiometer to the patient's earphones. The task of discriminating the sentences presented is made more difficult by distorting the speech signal or by adding a competing speech signal to the sentences. This competition can be added either to the same ear as the sentence or to the contralateral ear.

Jerger et al. (1968, 1972) found dramatic evidence of the profound effects central auditory lesions can exert on speech discrimination ability. In a study of a sixty-two-year-old male with bilateral temporal lobe insult when given the SSI test with a competing message added to the ipsilateral left ear, resulted in extreme difficulty in the patient's speech intelligibility of the test sentences. It appears that patients with unilateral temporal lobe disorders must be presented with rather difficult listening tasks before impaired speech intelligibility is shown. In patients with bilateral temporal lobe defects, however, the effect on speech discrimination ability is profound and may be demonstrated even under the easiest of listening conditions.

It would be of more than passing interest to see the effects of the

SSI test procedure with children with MBD since their defects more probably are due to more subtle lesions of the brain stem (most likely the reticular formation) rather than more gross lesions of the temporal lobe. Perhaps these children would most likely exhibit speech discrimination problems when given a competing message at the ipsilateral ear as the synthetic sentences. Allowances would, however, have to be made for those children with visual perceptual problems who might have difficulty scanning the ten sentences quickly in order to identify the one heard.

Perhaps, as we become more sophisticated and precise in our diagnosis of MBD, we will be able to differentially diagnose the disorder among three possible etiologies: (1) actual trauma and/or damage to specific areas of the CNS, (2) maturational delay in CNS development and functioning, and (3) neuroendocrine disorders resulting in incomplete impulse conduction either along the axon or across the synapse.

Basic equipment employed by an audiologist for auditory perceptual testing might include (1) a sound-treated room, (2) a dual-channel clinical audiometer complete with speech unit, phonograph and stereo tape deck, (3) dual stereo speakers in the subject test room, and (4) a one-way mirror so that the listener is truly in an *auditory isolated* situation with few visual distractions. Other equipment might include a variety of masking noise units and high- and low-pass speech filters. The sound-treated room should be set up to incorporate both sound-field and earphone test conditions.

Chapter 5

THERAPEUTIC CONSIDERATIONS

$\mathbf{A}$ THERAPEUTIC rationale should be based on auditory developmental norms and levels of auditory experience (see Tables I and II). The diagnosis should establish the level at which the child is functioning auditorily as opposed to how he should be functioning according to his age group. After the child's level of auditory perceptual ability has been established, a good rule of thumb is to begin therapy at one level lower than his established level. Since a strong auditory experiential backlog must be established, it is always better to review what we *suppose* the child has already established. This *going back* might also fill in the gaps in the child's perceptual disability that the diagnostic testing did not uncover.

Before any therapeutic considerations it is important to heed Wunderlich's (1971) caution to provide as much freedom to the child as possible so that he may know and become one with his environment:

> As parents and teachers, we must jealously find a way to provide freedom for little tykes — freedom of thought, expression, and movement! Little folks who are bottled up, contained, and regimented are apt to explode in adolescence, or they may wither in contrite acceptance of society's dicta. The provision of vast freedom within wide peripheral guidance limits is probably more important for children than any particular curriculum of instruction.

The main areas of therapeutic consideration are diagrammed in Figure 9.

AWARENESS

In order to increase awareness of sound, attention span and consistency of response the child must become aware of the *sound*

82

and *no sound* conditions. Before beginning any remediation for auditory perception, the environment in which the therapy is to take place must be controlled to insure a low ambient noise level and no distracting visual objects (including the clothing and other objects worn by the therapist and/or teacher). For some very distractible children, therapy in a sound-treated room may be the only answer until they become capable of coping with environmental sounds and distracting visual stimuli.

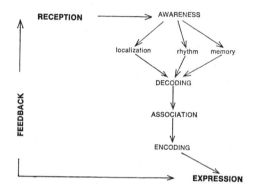

Figure 9. Diagram of auditory areas for therapeutic consideration.

Active manipulation of objects in the environment is encouraged. Toy animals that produce sounds are useful. The teacher encourages the child to listen. Later on, animal, truck, whistle and bell sounds can be recorded on a tape and played as the child is asked to point to the animal or object associated with the sound. Sound-to-object training should also cover cooking, traffic and recreation sounds. Emphasis should be placed on ear training whereby the child raises his hand or otherwise indicates that he can identify the desired sound from others made by the teacher. In speech awareness games, children can whisper instructions in one another's ears and follow through with the appropriate action. Another indicated technique is listening with telephones or walkie-talkies. The old game, "Simon Says," is still one of the best listening games for speech awareness.

Wunderlich (1971) tells us that the child should be encouraged to positive exploration of his environment with these words:

If one absolutely limits the possibilities for actions of a young child — by placing him in a large black box for six months — the child will then have to choose behavior only from those choices that are presented to him. Children have a basic urge to explore their environment and to be involved in their surroundings. They seek stimulation; they shun boredom. If the child is thus delimited but not coerced, he will choose a positive behavior pattern from the positive behavior patterns that are offered and allowed. The child detesting boredom will find stimulation in positive behavior if negative behavior is not allowed. The child will enjoy and seek positive behavior when it is reinforced with attention from a loved one and when the negative behavior is denied and/or ignored. Not only will the child choose a course of positive action but he will endow it with his own individual stamp if he is not made to conform to a mold. Then, the child becomes embued with the excitement of involvement and the thrill of originality, within the framework of supervised delimitation.

Barry (1961) approaches awareness training as a three-phase process: (1) awareness of gross sounds whereby a motor response is solicited to frequency differences in the sound of a bell, drum, whistle and horn; (2) awareness of finer sounds whereby beads are dropped into a tin, pebbles are rattled in a box, coins are jangled, a spoon is stirred in a cup; and (3) awareness of voice and speech whereby the child gives a motor response to digits, words, phrases and nonsense syllables. In the *Ithaca City Schools Perceptual Evaluation and Training Program* (by Dyer, Schramm, and Parsons), environmental sounds from the Peabody Record Kit No. 3 are presented. Next, sounds of musical instruments are given. Finally, taped stories containing environmental sounds are played and the children are asked to identify the sounds by naming the sounds, naming them in order of occurrence, and by classifying the sounds as to their location in the environment. Another interesting activity contained in this program is the presentation of different substances which are shaken in a tin (rice, sugar, cereal, salt). Identification of the substances is made by their sound in the tin and by their different tastes (gustatory stimuli).

LOCALIZATION

Localization training is best accomplished in a sound-treated room with a twin stereo speaker unit. Such games, however, as "turn to the sound," "hide and seek" and "find the sound" can be played in most classroom settings. It is best to have the child close his eyes while seeking the sound source. Gross body movements toward the sound source and following the sounds with the head and the fingers are suggested techniques.

RHYTHM

Kephart (1960) points out that information is kept classified and organized through rhythm being imposed upon auditory stimuli. Many difficulties with auditory memory span and temporal ordering of series information are due to weakness in establishing and/or maintaining rhythm patterns and problems in detecting the inflectional patterns of language.

Rhythm training incorporates the integration of auditory, kinesthetic and tactual rhythms. Unilateral rhythm tasks should be stressed first. The child is instructed to follow and maintain the rhythm pattern on a drum or similar object as established by the teacher. Variations in rate of beats (slow-fast, constant, 1 through 3 stage rhythms) should be imitated by the child. Foot tapping to the rhythm of the beats can also be stressed.

Bilateral rhythms may be learned after the child has established rhythm patterns on one side of the body. Emphasis is placed on beating out rhythms with both hands and/or feet. Alternating rhythms of equal phase between beats and of equal duration on drums or table tops are taught. The rhythm should alternate consistently (R-L-R-L or L-R-L-R) until the desired rhythm pattern is reproduced. More complicated rhythm patterns may be taught as the child progresses.

The rhythm patterns of language are stressed by particular inflectional patterns being superimposed on simple phrases and sentences. These same inflectional and rhythmic patterns can be varied and the cadence of the sentences altered to make sure the words are understood by the child.

Wunderlich (1971) feels that rhythmic ability indicates the child's ability to perform a motor act, then interrupt or change his action, and then return to a performance on time without being too early or too late. Rhythm, therefore, can be an indices of the flexibility of the child's inner controls. He can turn off and turn on in a periodic way.

MEMORY

Memory is the active comparison, elaboration and modification of input with previous inputs already experienced (Barr, 1971). Auditory memory is essential for language development, i.e. retention of sound sequences within words and of words within sentences. The teacher can combine memory exercises with those used to teach rhythm: (1) the child is instructed to tap on the table or clap his hands the same number of times and at the same intervals as the teacher, (2) the teacher has the child indicate by symbols associated with a sound or produce the actual figure corresponding to the number of sounds heard, and (3) the teacher plays tapes of various sounds several times in a set sequence and then on a replay has the child anticipate and identify each sound by pointing out in a picture or drawing the object which is going to produce the next sound. Advanced phonic association activities can be introduced later on. Some procedures involve the use of alphabet cards while asking the child, "What is the sound of this letter?" and the use of picture cards while asking the child "What sound does the name of this picture begin with?"

Story repetition is an important part of memory activities. As a short and simple story is related, have the child tell the general idea of the story. Later on, records and tapes of stories of longer length may be employed. Long-term recall days or weeks later can be stressed.

The Initial Teaching Alphabet (i/t/a). This approach to the teaching of reading began in Great Britain around twelve years ago, and around eight years ago in the United States. This tool for the initial teaching of reading is based on a carefully-designed phonemic alphabet. Imperfections are carefully built in to facilitate the transition from i/t/a to the traditional orthography. The i/t/a has forty-four symbols, each representing one phoneme (or sound) in the English language. Twenty-four of the symbols are traditional, fourteen are augmentations which closely resemble two familiar letters joined together, with the remaining six being special symbols. Once the child has learned these symbols and the sounds they represent, he can read any word written in i/t/a and write any word he can pronounce. In using the conventional alphabet, there are more than two thousand variations in the way the twenty-six symbols can be used to make the forty-odd sounds of English speech. These two thousand visual patterns are reduced to fewer than ninety patterns with the i/t/a (Downing, 1962).

This i/t/a approach is employed by Rampp (1972) at Memphis State University's Speech and Hearing Center with children with auditory perceptual disturbances. The primary reason for its success there is that the symbols are constant and never change; therefore, once the vowels and consonants have been learned, the child can read. This gives positive, early success to a child who has usually failed in his early attempts to read.

DECODING, ASSOCIATION, ENCODING

Once the child has learned to distinguish gross sounds he must learn fine differences between sounds in the environment and in speech. Decoding is the process of extracting meaning from auditory stimuli. This process can also be described as auditory discrimination and/or auditory receptive understanding. To correctly identify sounds and words, the child must be able to distinguish whether sounds or words are the same or different, and he must be able to distinguish in which part of the word — initial, medial or final — he hears a particular sound. He must also learn to discriminate similar environmental sounds and the qualities of voice inflection that reflect emotions. Barry (1961) stresses a four-phase therapeutic approach for teaching discrimination: (1) discrimination of gross sounds, (2) discrimination of finer sounds, (3) discrimination of voice and speech patterns, and (4) discrimination of musical instruments. Association is the internal manipulation of symbols and concepts. Encoding is the ability to express ideas in words. These three interdependent central processes of decoding, association and encoding combine to become the motor act of expression (output). Therapeutic approaches for these three processes center aound teaching words as meaningful units, vocabulary building and teaching the parts of speech.

Meaningful Units

If the child is taught to discriminate as to what means what, we are teaching him meaningful units. His understanding is best insured by reducing the amount of language used to give directions or explanations; by isolating key words; by timing the word with the visual symbol; by relating sound to object and word to experience (simultaneity); and by remembering that repetition is required for all learning, but more is necessary for children with auditory perceptual disorders.

Wunderlich (1970) says a movement act should be expected in each learning task:

> A performance (movement) act in *each* learning task for each child, as part of the daily curriculum! Too often the child is expected to perform only on a test! He should be expected to perform, do, and act in *all* subjects, day by day. It is not too much to expect homework from first or second-graders as long as it is brief. The point is to develop study habits and to get in there with some kind of performance work! Doing is knowing; doing is growing. In early grades, performance tasks might be assigned three days out of five, or some such scheme. For example, hearing a word, saying a word, *and* writing the word or constructing the word out of letters, or rearranging the word is desired. See, say, and write should be a routine.

Vocabulary and Parts of Speech

In vocabulary building, words are meaningful only when the child has the experience with which they are associated. Environmental exploration, field trips and tours should provide meaningful experiences. Instruction should concentrate on teaching meaningful words. Work on isolated sounds or nonsense syllables should depend on the amount of language the child has as well as the nature and extent of the auditory perceptual problem. Words having unlike or contrasting sounds should be taught first. Thereafter, like-sounding words which require finer auditory discrimination should be taught. Words should be considered as concepts, i.e. representations of ideas and feelings, in addition to their mere representations of objects.

In teaching parts of speech, deal first with nouns, naming objects represented and using freely facial expressions and gestures for emphasis. Thereafter, teach nouns as concepts together with their general and specific meanings, e.g. my mommy versus a mommy. Learning should progress from the feel to the sound and sight of the object, from the word for the object to its physical description.

Teach verbs for physical action, e.g. walk, run, skip, as much as possible by actual demonstration. Tactual, kinesthetic and visual feedback should help dramatically to relate the action to its identifying verb. The child must also learn to associate certain experiences within the temporal frame of reference. This is achieved linguistically by stressing the tenses of verbs with the concept of time and its passage.

Adjectives which describe and limit objects and experience must be taught with nouns or pronouns. Adjectives which relate to auditory experience should be stressed. Some adjectives stimulate the child's feelings and emotions for others. Their use is extrovertive, turning the child away from his usual preoccupation and concern with self to care and consideration for others. Before this can happen, however, he must learn the words that describe how others feel.

Prepositions by definition denote position in space. This

concept must be taught as a spatial relationship of one object(s) to another. These relationships or relative positions must also be constantly varied so that the child does not form a rigid idea of the positional concept. See Table VI for the Language Guide for Parents.

TABLE VI

LANGUAGE GUIDE FOR PARENTS*

1. Encourage your child to talk to you and take time to talk to your child.
2. Try to give him your undivided attention for at least a short period of time every day.
3. Let him tell you what he did, what he said and how he did it.
4. Ask him questions and encourage him to speak.
5. Listen to his ideas.
6. Answer his questions.
7. Reward him with verbal praise (that's good — you did well).
8. Make your child alert to sounds around him.
9. Identify sounds for your child.
10. Ask him what he thinks about matters which he can understand.
11. Name things for your child — help him to call things by their right names.
12. Help him to look at pictures and describe what he sees.
13. Help him to make up stories about pictures.
14. Tell him stories, fairy tales and nursery rhymes.
15. Stimulate your child to speak. You may want to put magazine pictures on the wall or give him objects to talk about.
16. Help your child to listen to the sounds around him and identify them (the ring of the phone, the television, the pots and pans, the water, the door slamming, the window closing, the clapping of hands).
17. You can play a game with your child — you make sounds and have him tell you what he has heard.
18. Take your child for a walk and talk about the things you see and hear.
19. While you're cooking, talk to your child about the foods you are making and the things you are doing.
20. On a trip to the grocery store, tell your child what you're buying — name the foods for your child. Do the same thing in any other store.
21. Whenever you go any place with your child, try to talk to him about where you are and what you see, hear and do.
22. Help your child to notice the things in his environment. Point out things to him, and perhaps even play a game of counting how many different things he sees or how many of one thing he sees.
23. Take every opportunity to talk to your child!

*From OPERATION: MOVING AHEAD, TITLE I PROJECT, PRINCE GEORGE COUNTY PUBLIC SCHOOLS, UPPER MARLBORO, MARYLAND.

REMEDIAL AND DEVELOPMENTAL PROGRAMS

The reader is directed to the following detailed developmental programs:

The Remediation of Learning Disabilities (1967) by Robert Valett. Under the "Perceptual-Motor Skills" section of this program the following auditory areas are considered: (1) auditory acuity, (2) auditory decoding, (3) auditory-vocal association, (4) auditory memory, and (5) auditory sequencing.

Aids to Psycholinguistic Teaching (1969) by Wilma Jo Bush and Marian Taylor Giles is another detailed remedial text. In the area of audition, programs in auditory reception, association, sequential memory and integrative techniques are presented in developmental sequence for grades one through eight.

Auditory Perception Training (APT) by Willette, Jackson, and Peckins (1970). The APT program is designed to present five areas of auditory perception sequentially, each area containing three levels of activities: (1) auditory memory, (2) auditory motor, (3) auditory figure-ground, (4) auditory discrimination, and (5) auditory imagery. These activities are designed for students with auditory perceptual problems because of minimal brain dysfunction as well as for those students in reading readiness programs.

Auditory Discrimination in Depth (ADD Program) by Charles and Patricia Lindamood (1969). The ADD Program is structured for students of all ages and develops the auditory skills basic to reading, speaking and spelling. The program can be used both developmentally and remedially. The following two levels of the program may be used with preschool and kindergarten children. At level one the child is introduced to selective listening and discriminates between differing sounds. Level two may be referred to as the *oral-aural level*. At this level the students learn to associate orally consonants and vowels according to the way formed in the process of enunciation (oral motor-kinesthetics). Next, the students manipulate colored blocks to group and identify the order of sounds in sequences. At the *sound-symbol level* the students relate letters and diphthongs to their sounds. A series of exercises and games with playing cards, one for each letter, emphasize left-to-right orientation, position in space, starting

and stopping points, order and sequence, and responses to auditory and visual cues. At the *symbol encoding or spelling level* the
student represents oral patterns by manipulating letter-symbol
titles and by writing down their patterns. Emphasis at this level is
placed on sound-to-label-to-symbol integration. The final level is
symbol decoding or reading. At this level the student translates
the letter patterns into the patterns of oral reading.

Sound/Order/Sense (SOS) by Eleanor Semel (1970). This is a
two-year auditory perception program which develops auditory
skills through 160 daily lessons. Level I is used for first graders,
and level 2 is started when the first level is completed. In the SOS
program, children are taught to listen for the sounds that comprise speech, the order or sequence of sounds in words and words
in groups, and the attributes (sense) that give meaning to words.
The remedial SOS program is designed for children with auditory
perceptual problems who require more intensive practice than is
available in the developmental program.

Kottler (1972) presents procedures and sample activities for
both identifying and rehabilitating children with auditory-
perceptual disorders related to sound localization, sound discrimination and sound sequencing. He discusses each of these
three areas in terms of the learning difficulties involved, prerequi-
site skills and whether tests are available to assess each perceptual
area. Class activities and games designed to train students in each
auditory perceptual skill are discussed. Activities for sound localization progress in difficulty from stationary child to sound, to
stationary child and moving sound, to moving child and stationary sound. Sound discrimination activities include matching
matching sounds, contrasting sounds (loud vs. soft, long vs.
short, fast vs. slow, high vs. low), and figure — ground discrimination. Sound sequencing activities are designed to emphasize
motor sequencing, following directions in sequence, and vocabulary of locations.

In the *Handbook of Auditory Training* by Cora Lee Reagan
(1973), a comprehensive program is presented which is designed
as a guide for training children with auditory perceptual dysfunctions. The tasks are arranged in sequential order so that gross
auditory discriminations may be mastered prior to the more

refined discrimination tasks. The tasks are designed to develop not only auditory perceptual ability, but the perceptual functions of visual-motor, tactile-kinesthetic and social-emotional areas as well.

Auditory Perceptual Disorders and Remediation by Bernice E. Heasley (1974). Auditory perceptual training lessons are offered in graduated degrees of difficulty, length of lesson time and number of processes to be introduced. The remediation tasks require no expensive equipment or materials.

See Table VII for How Parents May Contribute to Reading Development.

TABLE VII

HOW PARENTS MAY CONTRIBUTE TO READING DEVELOPMENT*

1. Maintain a relaxed, comfortable atmosphere at home where each child is made to feel important and wanted.
2. Give children plenty of experience — take them to the zoo, fire house, farm, historic spots, etc.
3. Be enthusiastic about school and school activities.
4. Give children a chance to talk about themselves and their interests.
5. Answer your children's questions in a simple, direct manner.
6. Praise your child for his accomplishments.
.7. Develop a feeling of independence by giving him responsibility.
8. Encourage your child to associate with other children.
9. Interest your child in things in which he should be interested.
10. Teach your child correct names of persons and things. Help him to associate people and places.
11. Let children see you reading with enjoyment.
12. Provide materials similar to those in school — paste, paper, paint, scissors, etc.
13. Insist that children know how to follow directions and pay attention.
14. Show your children that books aren't the only kind of reading. Magazines, menus, letters, road signs, etc., are other sources.
15. Follow your child's progress in school with interest, but do not burden him with minute questions about his activities.
16. Provide a daily paper and interesting magazines.
17. Help children to select a good balance of educational and recreational television programs, radio programs, movies and books.
18. Visit the school often for an objective report of your child's progress.
19. Get your child a library card and encourage him to use it.
20. Provide a quiet place for study.
21. Have periodic physical check-ups to insure that your child is in good health.

*From OPERATION: MOVING AHEAD, TITLE I PROJECT, PRINCE GEORGE COUNTY PUBLIC SCHOOLS, UPPER MARLBORO, MARYLAND.

UNIMODAL VS. BIMODAL PRESENTATION
(Sensory Integration)

When faced with a novel learning situation, Gaeth (1967) says that the child uses only one modality, and the single modality used is the one with the highest degree of redundancy. He further suggests that a multisensory stimulus presentation constitutes two learning tasks that must be separated for unisensory learning to occur. Thus, improvements in new learning situations employing bimodal presentation occur not from the integration of simultaneous bimodal stimulation, "but from the integration of rapidly alternating unimodal stimulation."

In light of Gaeth's findings, material should be presented initially for discrimination through the sensory channel in which an attempt is being made to improve perception, then through the alternate channel. Thus, unisensory presentation followed by bimodal presentation — e.g. auditory cues, then visual cues combined. When presenting the auditory cues, we should ask the child to listen, identify the sound and repeat it several times following the initial presentation of the auditory model. In this way feedback of the child's own speech is provided by his own repetitions of the sound and by recording it on a tape recorder for further playback. Mirror practice can be added to the visual cues in order that the child can see the way in which he produces sounds and becomes aware of the motor-kinesthetic sensations which arise from their production.

The ideas contained in Gaeth's data still await further examination; however, it would seem appropriate in a therapeutic sense not to overload the system of the child with MBD with too much information presented to too many sensory modalities. Common sense would dictate that information first be directed to the system under remediation, and then to another modality for multisensory integration of the input.

Recent research by Schlondorff and Tegtmeier (1973) lends support to Gaeth's unimodal presentation theory by pointing to the developmental difficulties incurred with unisensory auditory presentation with normal children ages five to thirteen years. In their study of the development of dichotic speech intelligibility, they found that the younger children suppressed information coming from one of the ears; even five-year-olds were capable of doing so. They concluded that complete mastery of the ability for dichotic selective listening is only attained at puberty.

It appears that while young children possess much functional central nervous system plasticity, the very existence of such plasticity allows for easy overloading of these CNS modalities by multisensory stimulation. Children with MBD obviously require still greater therapeutic planning in that they present still greater learning problems than normal children.

Universal agreement on the unimodal-then-bimodal approach is not to be found. Gaeth, it must be remembered, is directing his approach mainly to the remediation of the deaf.

A group of children with learning disabilities were matched by Ayres (1972) with a control group for degree and type of sensory integrative dysfunction. Her statistical analyses suggest that the greater improvement in academic scores of the experimental groups over the control groups were probably related to enhanced sensory integration due to an intervention program. This program provided vestibular stimulation (balancing tasks), tactile stimulation (in order to lower the level of excitation of the reticular formation), proprioceptive stimulation through muscle and joint receptors, manipulatory puzzles with language providing the usual means of communication, but no language skill training per se was given.

Ayres proposes that these results indicate that carefully-controlled sensory input through the vestibular and somatosensory systems enhances the capacity of the brain, particularly the brain stem, for intersensory integration between these modalities and the visual and auditory inputs that are a natural component, if only incidental, of the gross motor experience employed to elicit much of the stimuli. The mechanisms for these integrative processes are centered in the brain stem, thalamus and cerebral cortex. Ayres hypothesizes that normalization of postural mechanisms organized in the midbrain enables better interhemispheral communication at the cortical level. This postulate is derived from the obvious fact that many children with sensory integrative disorders have difficulty in the sensorimotor integration of the two sides of the body, and this problem is ameliorated when postural mechanisms are normalized through remedial therapy.

Chapter 6

CLASSROOM MANAGEMENT AND OTHER APPROACHES

SOUND classroom management of the perceptually handicapped child demands new and varied approaches. A current approach is based on a rationale for educational planning, utilizing ongoing diagnostic methodology during actual remediation. This approach is termed *diagnostic teaching*. Other classroom accommodations to help the teacher help the disabled child are presented as well as therapeutic approaches and considerations involving auditory sensitivity and motor training, auditory tracking, teaching listening skills, drug therapy and environmental considerations.

DIAGNOSTIC TEACHING

A common approach to total planning for remedying perceptual disorders involves the principle of progressive educational diagnoses. It should be obvious that standardized tests do not provide a complete picture of the disabled child as to etiology, prognosis, psychological ramifications, nor indicate the optimum course of rehabilitation. One reason is that the ongoing educational diagnosis involves diagnostic teaching based on the assumption that effective teaching of necessity incorporates the procedural sequences following in effective diagnostic procedures.

The learning situation of the child must be carefully controlled, giving special attention to the following areas of the diagnostic-remedial process: (1) educational planning based on information from standardized tests, e.g. intellectual and achievement levels and psychological functioning; (2) planning based on structured observation both in the home and school environments wherever possible; (3) planning based on the areas of

97

perceptual weakness, especially respecting the nature and extent, in educational terms, of the child's brain dysfunction; (4) planning for the proper instructional setting, conducive to both remedying the child's handicap and to the teacher's optimal functioning; (5) planning in regard to the temporal aspects of remediation, or how long must special educational training be continued to effect a desired change in the child; and (6) planning which contemplates other disabilities, e.g. possible hearing and/or visual pathology at the sensory end organs, speech problems, secondary emotional disorders.

CLASSROOM ACCOMMODATIONS

Clear speaking practices must be emphasized for teachers and parents of children with auditory perceptual problems. The following list of classroom suggestions are not complete in scope nor are they unique to this author. They represent what can be done to provide accommodations to help the child organize sensory data in the classroom environment.

1. Make sure the child is seated where he can best see and hear the teacher.

2. Experiment with various seating positions where the child will be free from excess stimulation and distractions.

3. Explain what is being taught while you are doing it by using the blackboard, pictures and other visual aids.

4. Remember to watch the child for signs of lack of concentration, understanding and attention.

5. Remember that when repetition does not work, rephrasing the material often does.

6. The teacher should know as much as possible about the extent of the auditory perceptual problems of her students in educational terms.

7. Speak clearly and naturally with no exaggeration of lip or facial movements. Gestures may be used freely unless they distract.

8. Emphasize differences in the phonemes of the language by having the child repeat the sounds and listen to them, not only as you say them but as he says them.

9. Reading programs should stress the basic sounds of the language using phonetic coding. Basic auditory skills should be taught when beginning the reading program.

10. Visual cues (colors, underlined words) should be used to aid the child in relating a specific phoneme to a visual stimulus.

11. Ask short simple questions and have the child repeat the question as part of his answer.

12. Isolate key words. Avoid multiple commands or directions and detailed instructions. Be sure the child understands the words used.

13. Allow and encourage the child to repeat instructions to himself and allow him to *tell* himself as he works. Subvocalization in reading should also be allowed until he is capable of eliminating this behavior.

14. Rhythm games, discrimination, sequencing, memory activities and singing should be stressed.

15. Alter the inflection, pitch, speaking rate and volume of your voice to emphasize key words and emotional content of the verbal message.

AUDITORY SENSITIVITY AND MOTOR TRAINING

In auditory sensitivity (imagery) training, a story (word pictures) is spoken to the child with his eyes shut. The child interprets the action of the story with the various body movements he feels appropriate. The ability to visualize and interpret an image from an auditory description is stressed.

In auditory motor training, simple directional commands are given at first, "Give me the chalk," "Go to the board and write your name," and so on. Progressively, the child learns correct responses to multidirectional commands, "Place your hands above your head, move them back and forth and then place them back at your sides." Following square dance directions by a caller which are superimposed on the dance music and interpreting the action depicted in songs while being sung are other commonly-used activities in auditory motor training. Body movement and auditory perception are stressed in the *Ithaca Schools Perceptual*

Evaluation and Training Program. In this program the children lie on the floor and perform the following movements to the beat of a drum: (1) turning the head completely to the right, then to the left; (2) raising the arms straight in front of the face and returning them to the floor; (3) raising the right leg up straight and returning it to the floor, then raising the left leg likewise; and (4) lifting the head to look at the toes and returning the head to the floor. A counting rhythm is established with the drum beat (or can with a plastic top) so children can establish a cadence of movement.

AUDITORY TRACKING

Auditory tracking techniques involve the following: (1) Pure tones are presented through an audiometer and the frequency of the tones is varied. Three equidistant lines are drawn on a sheet of paper and the child traces over the lower line when low frequency tones are presented, the middle line for midfrequency tones, and the top line for high frequency tones. (2) Have the child trace over three or more lines as the duration of the tones are varied from one-half to four seconds. The length of the lines should vary corresponding with the duration of the tones. (3) Have the child trace over a broad line for low intensity tones, a less broad line for tones of medium intensity, and a narrow line for high intensity tones. A piano may be substituted for the audiometer if need be. The perception of variations in frequency, duration and intensity is stressed (Kirk, 1969).

TEACHING LISTENING SKILLS

Perhaps the most neglected skill is teaching students developmental listening skills. In order to teach such skills, a logical, progressive program of activities and exercises must be initiated so that students can learn better to transform the process of receiving acoustical stimuli into the talent for listening, i.e. discriminating, analyzing and understanding. All classroom activities requiring oral language offer natural opportunities for teaching listening skills. Most of the suggested activities mentioned here are not particularly suited for children with minimal brain dysfunction but are intended for normal children's use in the ordinary classroom situation. It should be obvious that good listening is a learned skill not exclusively stressed for children with auditory perceptual problems. Perhaps some suggested activities can be modified for use with children having auditory perceptual problems.

The following are objectives in listening skills which all students should attain: (1) to learn that listening is a skill, (2) to increase awareness and alertness, (3) to ignore or adjust to distracting noise, (4) to recognize the emotion-laden words, (5) to recognize the speaker's theme and purpose, and (6) to use the advantage of quick thinking over rapid speech.

Importance of Listening Skills

Activities that stress careful listening to clearly spoken directions and keeping personal listening logs for future reference are used to impress on students the practical importance of gaining listening skills. A listening log should include a time record of each listening situation with a brief description of the nature of the speech heard or the sound listened to, and where the listening occurred. Listening tests which necessitate careful listening can be given with items such as, "Give the wrong answer to this question: Are you a citizen of the U.S.A.?" and "If the world is round, complete the following incorrectly: Dogs bury _____."

Increase Awareness and Alertness

Activities are emphasized which stress selective concentration on sounds of the environment (silent listening with eyes both opened and closed), listening while performing no other task, and trying not to anticipate what the speaker may say next but focusing attention on what he is actually saying. One helpful exercise is to divide the class into two groups. Give the two group leaders a complicated message which they are to whisper once to the next person, who in turn passes it on to the next, and so on. The last member of each group writes down the message and returns it to the teacher. Recognition is given to the group who has listened more accurately.

Learning to Ignore Distractions

Classes should be required to listen attentively despite the presence of competing noise. Have students deliver speeches while a television or radio is turned up loud, then quiz the other students as to the content of the speeches delivered.

Recognizing the Mood of the Speaker

Activities should be stressed which require students to make statements using a variety of moods (fright, confidence, anger, concern, uncertainty, jollity). Another suggested activity is to play records or tapes of formal speeches, ghost stories, poems, jokes and political talks. The students are then asked to explain how the speakers reveal their mood in the recording as reflected by their tone of voice and words used.

Learning to Recognize the Speaker's Purpose

Every form of communication has one or more specific purposes: to inform, to persuade, to amuse, to impress, to frighten. The major purpose of the speaker is revealed by his tone of voice, his style and by his choice of words. Recordings of famous speeches can be played to have the students tell the speaker's purpose, his method of delivery, intonation and word choice.

Recognizing the Central Theme

Usually able speakers state their theme or central idea with their opening words. It is therefore of paramount importance for the listener to pay full attention at the beginning of a speech. Usually later sections of a speech concern details and arguments supporting the speaker's central theme. Suggested activities include reading short stories and other selections and having the students suggest appropriate titles. Then ask the students to summarize the story in one sentence and give particulars of the story.

Learning to Take Notes

A most important aid to learning, especially from junior high through college, is skilled note making. Notes should summarize what is heard accurately but concisely so that they later stimulate memory of the entire discourse.

Preferring Speed of Thought to Speed of Speech

The average person can think four to five times more words per minute than he can speak. This differential can be used to the listener's advantage to anticipate probable points about to be made, to evaluate what is being said, and to summarize in one's mind what the speaker's principal points are.

Heasley (1972) mentions four main processes which appear critical in the development of listening skills in children. These deserve serious attention by the classroom teachers and/or the other specialists working with auditory perceptual disorders:

1. *Auditory Memory.* The auditory perceptual training should be directed toward both long and short-term memory. These kinds of exercises will implement improvement of auditory attention and attention span.

Among other techniques, auditory memory can be tested and extended by the teacher who allows a gradually increasing time lapse between the signal and the response (identification) by the child. This assists the child to remember for longer periods of time what the signal sounds like.

2. *Auditory Projection.* Many children will attend to sound at close range and/or in a one-to-one relationship. By gradually increasing the distance between the teacher, who presents the signal, and the listener, the ability to attend in stimuli at distances may be improved. Withdrawn children should profit from this type of training.

3. *Auditory Sequencing Ability.* This is closely related to auditory memory, but involves indentification of multiply-

presented sounds in the exact order in which they were presented. Children who fail in this processing ability will have
depressed language ability in general. They may verbalize freely
and inflect appropriately, but their productions may reflect
sound reversals or even a jargon-like quality.

Teachers can help a child with sequencing problems by presenting two gross, unlike sound instrument signals which the
child is assisted to identify in correct order. The number of
sounds to be identified is gradually increased as the child gains
skill. The teacher gradually moves from non-speech sounds to
animal sounds (a transitional step to speech sounds), then to
vowels, syllables, words and sentences. This takes a long period
of time and may require the services of all concerned with the
child's learning: teacher, parents, and speech and hearing therapists.

4. *Auditory Separation Ability.* This process involves screening
out irrelevant stimuli in order to attend to and process the primary, or desired, stimuli. In the classroom situation, the primary message would be the lesson being presented.

The classroom teacher may help children with auditory separation problems by presenting familiar tasks in the presence of
various kinds of background sound at gradually increasing
levels of intensity. The child should be appropriately reinforced
for his success in ignoring the interfering stimuli.

Various kinds of background sounds in the school setting
may be recorded for this purpose. For example, the common
sounds of doors being opened and closed, shuffling feet, desks
being moved, bells, lunchroom and hall noise, public address
announcements, gym classes and band practice are representa-
tive of the kinds of public school sounds which often interfere
with pupils' attention. Were such sounds pre-recorded and used
at gradually increasing levels of intensity as the irrelevant
stimuli to be screened out in a given auditory perception
training exercise, they might create less of a diversion, generally.

In teaching language listening comprehension, Kellogg (1971)
describes the use of The Kellogg Listening Model. This model is
organized on three perceptual levels — acuity, discrimination and
comprehension. Kellogg says that during the application of this
model "a listener needs to mentally ask himself questions at four

levels as he is listening or after he has listened. These questions are Who, What, When, Where; Why and/or How; So What, So How."

The model can be explained step-by-step to children and practice given in its usage. No explanation is required by the teacher when it is applied to classroom discussion following stories or other material read to the class. Questions can simply proceed up the hierarchy of comprehension from data recall to data application.

DRUG THERAPY

The child with MBD may benefit from psychotropic (psychoactive) drug therapy (Millichap, 1968, and Cott, 1971). Psychoactivating drugs may induce a soothing effect which may ameliorate those behavioral manifestations which make remediation difficult. Wunderlich (1970) mentions that many nonadapting children in school and society have what he calls a "neuro-allergic syndrome." He outlines the following treatment schedule:

1. Nutritional
   a. Change existing diet in some way
   b. Vitamin and mineral therapy in "balanced" regimen
   c. Megavitamins
2. Drug Therapy
   a. Antihistamine
   b. Corticosteroids
   c. Stimulants such as amphetamines (methylphenidate)
   d. Other psychoactive agents such as tranquilizers (thioridazine, chlordiazeparide, chlorpromazine, diphenhydramine and reserpine) and anticonvulsants (diphenzlhydantoin and Primidone)
3. Allergic desenitization
4. Environmental (dust and pollen elimination, sometimes by use of an electrostatic precipitating air cleaner)

Wunderlich (1971) explains his corticosteroid regimen as follows:

> The dosages of corticosteroids given to children varies with the individual. One has to start out with a particular dose derived from experience, and then modify this upwards or down-

wards. The dexamethasone preparation that I am using contains ½ mg. per tsp. and I often start out with ½ mg. or one tsp. twice daily, sometimes elevating this dose and sometimes diminishing it.

Very often I find that it is possible to get along with a homeopathic type of dose, and for this regimen I am using one to four drops of the dexamethasone elixir, that is the same strength preparation as noted previously, and then decreasing this as soon as possible. In other words, what I do is give a certain amount, watch for the therapeutic effect that I want, and as soon as I get it I back away from that dosage and try to maintain the lowest possible dose that gives the positive therapeutic effect, whether that be the elimination of hyperactivity, increase in auditory attention span, general attention span, etc.

After I find out the maintenance dose I begin to spread it out, and instead of giving it daily I would give it every other day, every third day, every fourth day, and so on, always trying to get away from the medication as fast as I can. Using this type of regimen and this type of treatment philosophy, it has been possible to treat most children quite successfully without running into the deleterious side-effects of corticosteroid therapy. Perhaps the most common side-effect seen is the precipitation of a respiratory tract infection or a skin infection, and for this reason I have also been using preventive antibiotic therapy on a very low maintenance type of regimen in addition to the corticosteroid.

The prescription of this medication is not by body weight but by the personal response of the individual child to the medication. I do not know of any way to judge the amount of drug that a child will need, except by the look of his tissues. Sometimes I can get a guide by the appearance of his conjunctivae, his nasal membranes and his pharyngeal lymphoid tissue.

The parents must be counselled that this medication is potentially harmful, although under careful supervision there is no reason for any harm to occur. I see the patients at least once a week initially, and gradually less often thereafter, and I counsel them to get in touch with me if at any time the child develops an infection or any untoward behavior.

Some children I have treated for as long as a year; others I treat for a number of weeks; some for a number of months; and some for just a number of days. Some children will get over their problem when you treat them for a while, and then take the drug away; others will relapse and need more courses of treatment. Very often I have used the megavitamin type of therapy for a balanced nutritional regimen to wean the children off the corticosteroids onto this type of nutritional regimen. This has been very helpful.

Silver (1971) notes that there are several drugs which alter the functioning of the reticular formation. It is well known that all children with MBD do not respond the same to drug therapy. Some of these drugs are clinically effective in minimizing the hyperactivity, distractibility and short attention span of children with MBD. Dextroamphetamine and methylphenidate hydrochloride are two of the most frequently used drugs. They, along with imipramine and magnesium premoline, all have one common function in the CNS, the potentiation of the effect of norepinephrine resulting in a relative increase in norepinephrine. Since an imbalance in the reticular formation results in a clinical syndrome, this syndrome is improved by drugs which increase the available central nervous system norepinephrine.

In his article, Doyle (1962) warns that the physician must avoid the blandishments of drug manufacturers and work with a half dozen types of psychotropic drugs. He should be thoroughly familiar with their dosage, potency and potential toxicity. The least toxic should be tried first with at least six types tried before giving up on drug therapy for a particular child. His final caution is that no medication should be used as a substitute for psychological, psychiatric or social help.

ENVIRONMENTAL CONSIDERATIONS

Classrooms should be designed to reduce the ambient noise level to allow for effective communication. The characteristics of a room that affect speech intelligibility are (1) the loudness level of the speech signal, (2) the reverberation time of the room, (3) the noise present, and (4) the shape of the room.

Loudness can be controlled by the shape and size of the room and by how the room has been acoustically treated. When a classroom has acoustically hard walls, floor and ceiling, the room is reverberant or live. The noise is reflected back and forth, and the students are immersed in the noise with the feeling that it comes from everywhere. If, however, the classroom is treated with absorbing materials, the noise reflected is reduced and the sound is coming directly from its source, for example, from the students themselves or from the air conditioners. When noise can be localized and reduced it is less annoying. The noise-absorbing materials used are acoustical tiles, carpets, padded seats and drapes. The rectangular-shaped rooms with flat or convex surfaces generally provide the best acoustical qualities. Too much acoustical absorption, however, can actually be a detriment to effective communication, with the room sounding dead (Van Riper and Irwin, 1958, and Kingsbury and Taylor, 1968).

Van Riper and Irwin (1958) explain what is meant by the term *percentage articulation*. As it suggests, this term refers to the percentage of syllables that will be heard correctly by the average listener. Percentage articulation can be measured by placing an individual or group with normal hearing in a room and presenting them a large number of nonsense syllables, such as ba, ka, fa, etc. Each syllable is produced separately and the listeners write down or otherwise indicate the syllables they think they hear. It is surprising to learn that even if a normal speaker is situated only three or four feet from a normal listener, and if that speaker speaks at an ideal loudness level (usually 60 to 70 dB above threshold), and if all extraneous effects of noise and room size and shape are eliminated, the average listener will hear only some 96 percent of the isolated sounds produced. Thus, a score of 96 becomes an ideal score to be pursued in the percentage articulation (P.A.) test for a large room.

Actually, a P.A. of 96 will be obtained in very few group listening situations. As far as auditoriums are concerned, a P.A. of 85 percent represents excellent listening; 75 percent, satisfactory; 65 percent, minimal; and anything below 65 percent is next to useless. These figures, it must be remembered, are for isolated nonsense syllables. Contextual speech would be heard with much greater accuracy. For example, if 70 percent of isolated syllables can be understood, perhaps up to 100 percent of contextual speech could be clear.

The following is the technique of computing the P.A. in an actual room:

$$P.A. = 96 \, K_L K_r K_n K_s$$

K_L is the factor of reduction of loudness: K_r, the factor or reduction for reverberation; K_n, the factor of reduction for noise; and K_s, the factor or reduction for the shape of the room. Thus, for each of these factors, a K unity of 1 represents a perfect score. If all four K's are 1, the final score will be 96, as can easily be established by substitution of the number factors in the above formula:

$$96 \times 1 \times 1 \times 1 \times 1 = 96$$

It is evident at a bad room feature for any of the above factors can destroy the listening usefulness of the room.

In relation to preferences in reverberation time, Van Riper and Irwin (1958) report that the shorter the reverberation time, the greater the speech intelligibility. They point out, however, that listeners do not always prefer the shortest reverberation time. In general, as the room gets larger in volume, listeners tend to prefer a longer reverberation time. Other things being equal, however, the shorter the period, the better the articulation. The preference for longer reverberation times is stronger for music than for speech among listeners.

Another important factor that determines reverberation time is the amount of energy that is reflected back. If, for instance, one is standing in the middle of an open field and speaks, almost none of the sound will be bounced back. The reverberation time will approach zero. If one talks in a room with the window open, two things will happen to the speech. Part of it will bounce back from the walls and part will travel out of the open windows. Thus, an open window can be regarded as a perfect absorbent — it gives back no sound. Obviously, other materials are not as absorbent as an open window. The coefficient of absorption of certain materials is the ratio of the absorption produced by it to the absorption of an equal area of open window. Thus, acoustic engineers have computed, usually for a frequency of 512 Hz, the coefficients of absorption of various materials.

ENVIRONMENTAL STRESS

Wunderlich (1971) finds that a fundamental process is evident as we view the rapid rate of change and high level of activity that occurs in early childhood. "The more active an organism is, the more contacts he has with his environment. The more contacts he has, the more adaptations he must make to that environment." Obviously, if the child must make frequent and varied adaptations to his environment, the chances are greater of him making some adaptations that are unfavorable to himself. Therefore, greater activity increases vulnerability and the necessity for more problem solving. But what of those children who must make frequent adaptations to meet the demands of an ever changing and novel environment?

Toffler (1970), in his best selling book, *Future Shock,* puts forth the thesis that there are discoverable limits to the amount of change that the human organism can cope with, and that by endlessly accelerating change without first ascertaining these limits we may well be submitting masses of people to demands they simply cannot tolerate. The state of overstimulation these individuals are thrown into is what Toffler terms "future shock." Future shock is defined as the distress, both physical and psychological, arising from an overloading of the human organism's physical adaptive systems and its decision-making processes. More simply put, "future shock is the human response to overstimulation."

A novel change in the stimuli presented to the human organism results in what experimental psychologists call an *orientation response* (see Chapter 2 for a discussion of reflexive hearing). The orientation response (OR) is a complex massive systemic operation which affects the entire body: photochemical changes occur in the retina, hearing becomes more acute, involuntarily we use our muscles to direct the sense organs toward the incoming stimuli, the pupils of the eyes dilate, general muscle tone rises, changes occur in brain wave patterns, palms sweat, breathing and heart rate alter, etc. These changes occur everytime we perceive novelty in our environment, and the OR occurs literally thousands of times in the course of a day as changes occur in our environment.

Apparently, the OR is triggered when the new stimuli arriving at the brain do not match the other neural models in the cortex. If, however, the stimuli match other stored neural models in similarity, the cortex inhibits the activity of the reticular formation and the OR does not occur. Each OR takes its toll in wear and tear on the body. As the neural system responds to novel stimuli, its synaptic vesicles discharge adrenalin and noradrenalin which in turn trigger a partial release of the body's stored energy.

Situations which cannot be handled by a quick burst of energy, as released by the OR, necessitate a larger, more sustained reaction called the *adaptive reaction*. While the OR is primarily nervous system (brain stem) mediated, the adaptive reaction is heavily dependent upon the endocrine system and the hormones secreted into the bloodstream. One of the major substances secreted by the pituitary gland is ACTH, which goes to the adrenal glands and causes them to manufacture corticosteroids which in turn serve to speed up body metabolism. Thus, the adaptive reaction provides a much stronger and sustained release of energy than the OR. A more dramatic term for the adaptive reaction is *stress*. The repeated firing of the OR and the adaptive reaction can overload the neural and endocrine system, causing perceptual stress which can be linked to other diseases and physical problems as well. In order to understand this syndrome, Toffler suggests that we pull together such scattered fields as psychology, neurology, communications theory and endocrinology. These different scientific disciplines can help us to more clearly understand human adaptation. Perhaps we should have a science of adaptation per se (adaptology?), with a systematic listing of the diseases of adaptation along with indications for remediation.

Perhaps we can consider children with MBD as the first casualties of perceptual stress in an "overcharged" society such as the United States. Since these children have a more restricted "adaptive range" due to their perceptual disorders, ever increasing rates of change and novelty carry with them ever increasing sensory bombardment, creating sensory overload. They respond by confusion, anxiety, irritability and withdrawal into apathy.

As we strive to control runaway technology, ever increasing rates of change in our society and attempt to shift education into the future tense, we must provide perceptual havens in which children with MBD might learn, grow and, yes, retreat when necessary. By becoming such a haven, the school would become a place actively sought out by the perceptually handicapped child, where learning becomes a positive means of coping with and adjusting to his environment.

SUMMARY

The capabilities of the human voice to articulate intelligible sound and the human ear to transmute and transmit such sound to the highly selective and complex central nervous system for comprehension and response are essential to effective speech communication. Because most social and intellectual life begins with popular understanding of the spoken word prior to our becoming literate, we may say, in a larger sense, the progress of our civilization depends on the widespread development and protection of these capabilities among the peoples of our world. Moreover, the aesthetic qualities of our lives enhanced initially by the beauty in our environment can also be increased by eliminating or suppressing sources of controllable noise and, whenever possible by improving the nature and lowering the levels of sound we cannot avoid.

In considering perception, it must be understood that input is not easily separated from output. This author has attempted, however, in the short span of this book to focus on the listening experiences of children which provide the foundation for language acquisition. Oral expression has therefore received less attention. In a strict neurological sense, cortical and subcortical systems do not lend themselves to arbitrary division, making for conveniently understanding separate functions of each. Coding sensory stimuli is a continuous process, and thus no portion of the coding process is autonomous or independent. The central nervous system should be viewed as a circular system with adaptive and projectional tracts which are multidirectional.

The early maturing receptive system of the infant for processing acoustical and linguistic input must receive, however, careful investigation as a topic apart from expression. To understand this need, we have only to consider the primacy of listening over speech in infant growth and communication. Friedlander (1970) points out that the infant's learning to listen is not a passive stage of development but a profoundly dynamic and energetic undertaking, requiring the highest active capabilities of the child in adapting to the challenges of his environment. The fact that this receptive process is covert and difficult to investigate only adds to the challenge which we as teachers, diagnosticians, therapists and researchers face.

REFERENCES

Abramovitz, A.: Devising a developmental test of auditory perception: Problems and prospects. *J S Afr Speech Hearing Assoc, 18*:11-22, 1971.

Adey, W. R.: Hippocampal theta rhythm and approach behavior. *Prog Brain Res, 27*:228, 1967.

Anderson, R. M., Miles, M., and Matheny, P.A.: *Communicative Evaluation Chart From Infancy to Five Years.* Cambridge, Educators Publishing Service, 1963.

Ayers, A.J.: Improving academic scores through sensory integration. *J Learn Disabil,* June-July, 1972.

Bancaud, J., Bloch, V., and Paippard, J.: Contribution EEG a L'etude des potentials evoques chez L'homme au niveau du vertex. *Rev Neurol, 89*:399-418, 1953.

Banquet, J. P.: EEG and meditation. *Electroencephalogr Clin Neurophysiol, 33*:449-455, 1972.

Banquet, J. P.: Spectral analysis of the EEG in meditation. *Electroencephalogr Clin Neurophysiol, 35*:143-151, 1973.

Barr, D. F., and Carmel, N. R.: Stuttering inhibition with live voice interventions and masking noise. *J Aud Res, 10*:59-61, 1970.

Barr, D. F.: The Audiologist's role in auditory perceptual disorders. Paper presented at the Florida Speech and Hearing Assoc. Convention, Tampa, March 1971.

Barr, D. F. : Le role de l'audiologiste dans les cas de troubles de perception auditive. *Revue De La Societe Francaise D'Etudes De Correction Auditive, 25*: June, 1973.

Barr, D. F.: A study of auditory perceptual disorders in children with reference to language learning. Ph.D. thesis, Patna University, 1974.

Barry, H.: *The Young Aphasic Child: Evaluation and Training.* Washington, Alexander Graham Bell Assoc. for the Deaf, 1961, pp. 6-37.

Bateman, B. D., and Schiefelbusch, R. L.: Educational identification, assessment, and evaluation procedures (Section II). *In Minimal Brain Dysfunction in Children,* Phase Two, U.S. Dept. of H.E.W., 1969.

Belmont, I., Birch, H.G., and Karp, E.: The disordering of intersensory integration by brain damage. *J Nerv Ment Dis, 141*: 410-418, 1965.

Benton, A. L., Sutton, S., Kennedy, J. A., and Brokaw, J. R.: The cross-modal retardation in reaction time of patients with cerebral diseases. *J Nerv Ment Dis, 135*:413-418, 1962.

Berger, H.: Uber das elektrenkephalogramm des menchen. *Arch Psychiatr*

Nervenkr, 87:527-570, 1929.

Berry, M. F.: *Language Disorders of Children: The Bases and Diagnosis.* New York, Appleton, 1969.

Birch, H. G., and Belmont, L.: Auditory-visual integration, intelligence and reading ability in school children. *Percept Mot Skills, 20*:295-305, 1965.

Birch, H. G., and Belmont, I.: Auditory-visual integration in brain damaged and normal children. *Dev Med Child Neurol, 7*:135-144, 1965.

Birch, H. G. and Lefford, A.: Intersensory development in children. *Monogr Soc Res Child Dev,* Vol. 28, 1963.

Blakemore, C. B.: Psychological effects of temporal lobe lesions in man. In *Current Problems in Neuropsychiatry.* Special Pub. No. 4, *Br J Psychiatry,* 1969, pp. 60-69.

Broadbent, D. E.: *Perception and Communication.* New York, Pergamon 1958.

Broverman, D. M., Klaiber, E. L., Vogel, W., and Kobayashi, Y.: Short-term versus long-term effects of adrenal hormones on behaviors. *Psychol Bull, 81* (10):672-694, 1974.

Bruner, J. S.: Neural mechanisms in perception. *Res Pub Assoc Res Nerv Ment Dis, 36*: 118-143, 1958.

Bush, W. J., and Giles, M. T.: *Aids to Psycholinguistic Teaching.* Columbus, Merrill, 1969.

Capute, A. J., Niedermeyer, E. F. L., and Richardson, F.: The electroencephalogram in children with minimal cerebral dysfunction. *Pediatrics, 41*: 1104-1114, 1968.

Chatterjee, S. C., and Datta, D. M.: *An Introduction to Indian Philosophy.* Calcutta Pr, 1968.

Chatterjee, S. C.: *The Nyaya Theory of Knowledge.* Calcutta U Pr, 1965.

Chomsky, N.: The formal nature of language. In E. Lenneberg (Ed.), *Biological Foundations of Language.* New York, Wiley, 1967.

Church, J.: *Language and the Discovery of Reality.* New York, Random, 1961.

Clements, S. D.: *Minimal Brain Dysfunction In Children: Terminology and Identification.* NINDS Monograph No. 3, U.S. Dept. of H.E.W., Bethesda, 1966.

Conrad, K.: Versuch einer psychologischen Analyse des Parietalsyndromes. *Monateschr Psychiat U Neural,* p. 84, 1932.

Cott, A.: Orthomolecular approach to the treatment of learning disabilities. *Schizophrenia,* 2nd quart, *3*(2): 95-105, 1971.

Critchley, M.: Speech and Speech-loss in relation to duality of the brain. In Mountcastle, V. (Ed.): *Interhemispheric Relations and Cerebral Dominance.* Baltimore, Johns Hopkins, 1962, pp. 208-213.

Curry, F. K. W.: A comparison of left-handed and right-handed subjects on verbal and non-verbal dichotic listening tasks. *Cortex, 3*:343-352, 1967.

Curry, F. K. W., and Gregory, H. H.: The performance of stutterers on dichotic listening tasks thought to reflect cerebral dominance. *J Speech Hear Res, 12*:73-82, 1969.

Datta, D. M.: *The Six Ways of Knowing.* Calcutta U Pr, 1972.

Davis, P. A.: Effects of acoustic stimuli on the waking brain. *J Neurophysiol,* 2:494-499, 1939.

Delgado, J. M.: Free behavior and brain stimulation. *Int Rev Neurobiol,* 6:349-449, 1964.

Denhoff, E., Hainsworth, P., and Hainsworth, M.: The child at risk for learning disorder. *Clin Pediatr, 11*:3, 1972.

Desmedt, J. E.: Neurophysiological mechanisms controlling acoustic input. In Rasmussen, Grant and Windle, William (Eds.): *Neural Mechanisms of the Auditory and Vestibular Systems.* Springfield, Thomas, 1960.

Douglas, R. J.: The hippocampus and behavior. *Psychol Bull, 67*:416-442, 1967.

Downing, J. A.: The i t a (Initial Teaching Alphabet) reading experiment. *The Reading Teacher, 18*:105-109, 1962.

Doyle, P. J.: The organic hyperkenetic syndrome. *J Sch Health, 8,* 1962.

Drew, A.: A neurological appraisal of familial congenital word-blindness. *Brain, 79*:440-460, 1956.

Dyer, S., Schramm, D., and Parsons, C.: *Ithaca City Schools Perceptual and Training Program* (undated manual), Ithaca, N.Y.

Evans, J.R.: Auditory and auditory-visual integration skills as they relate to reading. *The Reading Teacher, 22*:625-629, 1969.

Feldman, S., Todt, J. C., and Porter, R. W.: Effect of adrenocortical hormones and evoked potentials in the brainstem. *Neurology, 11*:109-115, 1961.

Friedlander, B. Z.: Identifying and investigating the major variables of receptive language development. Paper presented at the meeting for the Society for Research in Child Development, Santa Monica, Califor., March 1969a.

Friedlander, B. Z.: The effect of speaker identity, voice inflection, vocabulary, and message redundancy on infants' selection of vocal reinforcement, *J Exp Child Psychol, 6*:443-459, 1969b.

Friedlander, B. Z.: Receptive language development in infancy: Issues and problems, *Merrill-Palmer Q, 16*:7-51, 1970.

Gaeth, J.: Deafness in children. In McConnell, F., and Ward, P. (Eds.), *National Symposium on Deafness in Childhood.* Nashville, Vanderbilt U Pr, 1967.

Galambos, R.: Inhibition of activity in single auditory nerve fibers by acoustic stimulation. *J Neurophysiol,* pp. 287-303, Sept. 1944.

Gesell, A., and Amatruda, C. S.: *Developmental Diagnosis,* 2nd ed. New York, Hoeber Medical Div. Har-Row, 1967.

Getman, G. N.: Explorations into visual-auditory space, *Optometric Extension Program,* vol. *41*(12): 76, August 1969.

Ghosh, M.: *Paniniya Siksa.* Calcutta U Pr, 1938, pp. 72-73.

Graham, P., and Rutter, M.: Organic brain dysfunction and child psychiatric disorder. *Br Med J, 11*:695-700, 1968.

Grastyan, E.: The hippocampus and higher nervous activity. In Brazier, M. A. B. (Ed.): *The Central Nervous Sytem and Behavior,* New York, Josiah Macey, Jr. Foundation, 1959.

Grastyan, E.: The significance of the earliest manifestations of conditioning in the mechanism of learning. In Delafresnaye, J. F. (Ed.): *Brain*

Mechanisms and Learning. Oxford, Blackwell, 1961.

Gray, W.: *Standardized Reading Paragraphs.* New York, Bobbs, Psychological Corp., 1955.

Heasley, B. E.: Auditory perception and remediation. *Acta Symbolica, 3*(2):135-136, 1972.

Heasley, B. E.: *Auditory Perceptual Disorders and Remediation.* Springfield, Thomas, 1974.

Hebb, D. O.: *The Organization of Behavior,* New York, Wiley, 1949.

Henkin, R. I., McGlone, R. E., Daly, R., and Bartter, F. C.: Studies on auditory thresholds in normal man and in patients with adrenal cortical insufficiency: The role of adrenal cortical steroids. *J Clin Invest, 46:*429-435, 1967.

Henkin, R. I., and Daly, R. L.: Auditory detection and perception in normal man and in patients with adrenal cortical insufficiency: Effect of adrenal cortical steroids. *J Clin Invest, 47:*1269-1280, 1968.

Henkin, R. I.: The neuroendocrine control of sensation. In *The Second Symposium on Oral Sensation and Perception.* Springfield, Thomas, 1969.

Henkin, R. I.: The neuroendocrine control of perception. *Perception and Its Disorders.* Res. Publ. A.R.N.M.D., Vol. *48*(5):55-107, 1970.

Hughes, J. R.: Electroencelphalograph and learning. In Myklebust, Helmer R. (Ed.): *Progress In Learning Disabilities.* New York, Grune, vol. 1, 1968.

Hunter, I. M. L.: *Memory: Facts and Fallacies.* Baltimore, Penquin, 1957.

Jerger, J., Speaks, C., and Trammell, J.: A new approach to speech audiometry. *J Speech Hearing Dis, 33:*, 1968.

Jerger, J., Lovering, L., and Wertz, M.: Auditory disorder following bilateral temporal lobe insult: Report of a case. *J Speech Hearing Dis, 37,* 1972.

Kellogg, R. E.: Listening. In Lamb, P. (Ed.), *Guiding Children's Language Learning.* Dubuque, Wm. C. Brown, 1971.

Kephart, N. C.: *The Slow Learner in The Classroom,* Columbus, Merrill, 1960.

Kimmell, G. M., and Wahl, J.: *The STAP, Screening Test For Auditory Perception.* San Rafael, Academic Therapy Publications, 1969.

Kimura, D.: Cerebral dominance and the perception of verbal stimuli. *Can J Psychol, 15:*166-171, 1961.

Kimura, D.: Functional asymmetry of the brain in dichotic listening. *Cortex, 3:*163-178, 1967.

Kimura, D.: Left-right differences in the perception of melodies. *Q J Exp Psychol, 16:*355, 1964.

Kingsbury, H. E., and Taylor, D. W.: Guidelines for acoustical design of classrooms. *Sound and Vibration, 10:*17-29, 1968.

Kirk, R. D.: Auditory tracking techniques. *Auditory Receptivity Program.* Springfield, The Learning Center, American Int. College, 1969.

Kirk, S., McCarthy, J., and Kirk, W.: *Illinois Test for Psycholinguistic Abilities.* Urbana, U of Ill Pr, 1968.

Kottler, S. B.: The identification and remediation of auditory problems. *Acad*

Ther Q, 8(1):73-86, 1972.

Kurtz, D.: Automatic analyzer for screening inborn errors of metabolism. Workshop Resume, National Institute of Neurological Diseases and Blindness, May 1965.

Lenneberg, E.: *Biological Foundations of Language.* New York, Wiley, 1967.

Lindamood, C., and Lindamood, P.: *L.A.C. Test (Lindamood Auditory Conceptualization Test).* Boston, Teaching Resources, 1970.

Lindamood, C., and Lindamood, P.: *A.D.D. Program (Auditory Discrimination in Depth).* Boston, Teaching Resources, 1969.

Lindsley, D.: Common factors in sensory deprivation, sensory distortion, and sensory overload. In Solomon, P. *et al.: Sensory Deprivation.* Cambridge, Harvard U Pr, 1961.

Ling, A. H.: Dichotic listening in hearing-impaired children. *J Speech Hear Res, 14:*793-803, 1971.

Lovitt, T.C.: Assessment of children with learning disabilities. *Except Child, 34:*233-239, 1967.

Lumley, F. H., and Calhoun, S. W.: Memory span for words presented auditorily. *J Appl Psychol, 10:*733-784, 1934.

Luria, A. R.: Aspects of aphasia. *J Neurol Sci,* May/June 1965, pp. 278-287.

Luria, A. R.: *Higher Cortical Functions in Man.* New York, Basic, 1966.

Mark, H. J.: Psychodiagnostics in patients with suspected minimal brain dysfunction(s), Appendix B., *Minimal Brain Dysfunction in Children.* Public Health Service Publ. No. 2015, 1969, pp. 75-76.

McCandless, G.A.: Electroencephalic audiometry. In Rose, Darrell E. (Ed.): *Audiological Assessment.* Englewood Cliffs, P-H, 1971.

McGrady, H.: Language pathology and learning disabilities. In Myklebust, H. R. (Ed.): *Progress In Learning Disabilities.* New York, Grune, vol. 1, 1968.

Merifield, D. O.: The otolaryngologist and learning disabilities, *Arch Otolaryngol, 91,* 1970.

Millichap, J. G.: Drugs in management of hyperkinetic and perceptually handicapped children. *JAMA, 206:*1527, 1968.

Milner, B. L.: Psychological defects produced by temporal lobe excision. *Res Publ Assoc Nerv Ment Dis, 36:*244-257, 1958.

Milton, A. W.: Implications of short-term memory for a general theory of memory. *J Verb Learn Verb Behaviour,* 2:1-21, 1963.

Minckler, J.: *Introduction to Neuroscience.* Saint Louis, Mosby, 1972.

Moruzzi, G., and Magoun, H. W.: Brain stem reticular formation and activation of the EEG. *Electroencephalagr Clin Neurophysiol, 1:*455-473, 1949.

Muehl, S., and Kremenak, S.: Ability to match information within and between auditory and visual sense modalities and subsequent reading achievement. *J Educ Psychol, 57:*230-238, 1966.

Myklebust, H. R.: *Auditory Disorders in Children,* New York, Grune 1954.

Nauta, W. J. H.: Hippocampal projections and related neuronal pathways to the midbrain in the cat. *Brain, 81:*319-340, 1958.

Obrador, S.: Nervous integration after hemispherectomy in man. In Schaltenbrand, G., and Woolsey, C. (Eds.): *Cerebral Localization and Organization.* Madison, U of Wis Pr, 1964, p. 141.

Orton, S.: *Reading Writing and Speech Problems in Children.* New York, Norton, 1937.

Ounsted, C., Lindsay, J., and Norman, R.: *Biological Factors In Temporal Lobe Epilepsy.* London, Heinemann, 1966.

Papcun, G., Keashen, S., Terbeek, D., Remington, R., and Harshman, R.: Is the left hemisphere specialized for speech, language and/or something else? *J Acoust Soc Am, 55*(2):319-327, 1974.

Parnell, P., and Korzeniowski, R.: Auditory perception and learning (Part II). *Remedial Educ, 4*(4):20-22, 1972.

Penfield, W., and Roberts, L.: *Speech and Brain Mechanisms.* Princeton, Princeton U Pr, 1959.

Pond, D. A., and Bidwell, B. H.: A survey of epilepsy in fourteen general practices: Social and psychological aspects. *Epilepsia, 1*:285-299, 1960.

Pond, D. A.: Temporal lobe epilepsy in children. In *Current Problems In Neuropsychiatry.* Special Pub. No. 4, *Br J Psychiatry,* 1969, 82-86.

Poole, I.: Genetic development in articulation of consonant sounds in speech. *Elem Engl, 11*:159-161, 1934.

Prentky, J.: Minimal brain dysfunction in children. *J Spec Educ Ment Retard, 9*(1):14-20, 1972.

Rampp, D.L.: Auditory perceptual distrubances, In Weston, A. (Ed.): *Communicative Disorders: An Appraisal.* Springfield, Thomas, 1972.

Reagan, C. L.: *Handbook of Auditory Perceptual Training.* Springfield, Thomas, 1973.

Reynolds, E. H., Chanarin, I., Milner, G., and Matthews, D. M.: Anticonvulsant therapy, folic acid and vitamin B12 metabolism and mental symptoms. *Epilepsia, 7*:261-270, 1966.

Reynolds, E. H.: Schizophrenia-like psychoses of epilepsy and disturbances of folate and vitamin B12 metabolism induced by anticonvulsant drugs. *Br J Psychiatry, 113*:911-919, 1967.

Rimland, B.: *Infantile Autism.* New York, Appleton, 1964.

Roberts, D. R.: Schizophrenia and the brain. *J Neuropsychiatry, 5*:71-79, 1963.

Rose, J. E., Gross, N. B., Geisler, C. D., and Hind, J. E.: Some neural mechanisms in the inferior colliculus of the cat which may be relevant to localization of a sound source. *J Neurophysiol, 29*:288-314, 1966.

Rosenblith, J. F.: The Modified Graham Behavior Test for Neonates: Test-retest reliability, normative data and hypothesis for future work. *Biologic Neonatorum, 3,* 1961.

Rosenzweig, N.: A mechanism in schizophrenia: A theoretical formulation *Arch Neurol Psychiatry, 74*:544-555, 1955.

Rosner, J., and Simon, D.: *The Auditory Analysis Test: An Initial Report.* Pittsburgh, Learning Research and Development Center, University of Pittsburgh, 1970.

Rosner, J.: *The Rosner Perceptual Survey (RPS).* Working Paper 47. Pittsburgh, Learning Research and Development Center, University of Pittsburgh, 1969.

Roswell, F. G., and Chall, J. S.: *Auditory Blending Test,* New York, Essay Pr, 1963.

Routtenberg, A.: The two arousal hypothesis: Reticular formation and limbic system. *Psychol Rev,* 51-80, 1968.

Sanders, D. A.: *Aural Rehabilitation.* Englewood Cliffs, P-H, 1971.

Schlondorff, G., and Tegtmeier, W.: The development of dichotic speech intelligibility. *Z Laryngol Rhinol, 52*(1):28-31, 1973.

Schuell, H., Jenkins, J., and Jimenez-Pabon, E.: *Aphasia in Adults.* New York, HarRow, 1964.

Semel, E.: *Sound Order Sense.* Chicago, Follett, 1970.

Silver, L.: A proposed view on the etiology of the neurological learning disability syndrome. *J Learning Disabilities, 4,*(3):123-133, 1971.

Sinha, S. P.: The role of the temporal lobe in hearing. Master's thesis, McGill University, 1959.

Sklar, B., Hanley, J., and Simmons, W.: An EEG experiment aimed toward identifying dyslexic children. *Nature, 240*:414-416, 1972.

Symthies, J. R.: *The Neurological Foundations of Psychiatry.* Oxford, Blackwell, 1966.

Smythies, J. R.: Brain mechanisms and behavior. *Brain, 90*:697-706, 1967.

Smythies, J. R.: The behaviorial physiology of the temporal lobe. In *Current Problems In Neuropsychiatry.* Special Pub. No. 4, *Br J Psychiatry,* 9-15, 1969.

Smythies, J. R.: *Brain Mechanisms and Behaviour.* New York, Acad Pr, 1970.

Solley, C. M., and Murphy, P.: *Development of the Perceptual World.* New York, Basic, 1960, p. 18.

Staehelin, J. E.: Psychopathologie der Zwichen — und Millelhirn-Krankungen. *Schweiz Arch Neurol Psychiat, 53*:374-395, 1944.

Stevens, K. N., and Halle, M.: Remarks on analysis by snythesis and distinctive features. In Weiant Wathen — Dunn (Ed.): *Models For The Perception of Speech and Visual Form.* Cambridge, M.I.T. Pr, 1967.

Taylor, I. G.: Development of evoked responses in audiological diagnosis. *Sound, 2*:102-105, 1968.

Toffler, A.: *Future Shock.* New York, Random, 1970.

Tsunoda, T.: Contralateral shift of cerebral dominance for nonverbal sounds during speech perception. *J Aud Res, 3*:221-229, 1969.

Turner, E. A.: A surgical approach to the treatment of symptoms in temporal lobe epilepsy. In *Current Problems in Neuropsychiatry,* special pub. No. 4, *Br J Psychiatry,* 102-105, 1969.

Underwood, B. J.: The representativeness of rote verbal learning. In Melton, A. W. (Ed.): *Categories of Human Learning.* New York, Acad Pr, 1964.

Valett, R. E.: *The Remediation of Learning Disabilities,* Palo Alto, Fearon, 1967, Section 22-37.

Van Riper, C., and Irwin, J.: *Voice and Articulation*. Englewood Cliffs, P-H, 1958.

Wepman, J.: *Wepman Test of Auditory Discrimination*. Chicago, Language Research Associates, 1958.

Wepman, J.: Auditory discrimination in speech and reading. *Elementary School J, 60*:325-333, 1960.

Whitehead, A. N.: *The Aims of Education*. New York, MacMillian, 1929.

Witelson, S. F., and Pallie, W.: Left hemisphere specialization for language in the newborn. *Brain, 96*(3):641-646, 1973.

Willette, R., Jackson, B., and Peckins, I.: *Auditory Perception Training (APT)*. Chicago, Developmental Learning Materials, 1970.

Wunderlich, R. C.: Learning disorders — A developmental approach. *J Learning Disabilities, 1*:128-133, 1968.

Wunderlich, R. C.: *Kids, Brains and Learning*. St. Petersburg, Johnny Reads, 1970.

Wunderlich, R. C.: Personal Communication, 1971.

Wunderlich, R. C.: Developmental correlates in learning. *Acad Ther, 7*, 1971.

Zach, L., and Kaufman, J.: How adequate is the concept of perceptual deficit for education. *J Learn Disabil*, June-July, 1972.

SUGGESTED READINGS

Adler, S.: *The Non-verbal Child,* Springfield, Thomas, 1964.

Adler, S.: Pediatric psychopharmacology and the language-learning impaired child. *ASHA, 16*(6): 299-304, 1974.

Asimov, I.: *The Human Brain: Its Capacities and Functions.* HM, 1964.

Bakker, D. J., Smink, T., and Reitsma, P.: Ear dominance and reading ability. *Cortex, 9*(3): 301-312, 1973.

Bakker, D. J., and Satz, P. (Eds.): *Specific Reading Disability: Advances In Theory and Method.* Portland, Int'l Scholarly Book Serv., 1970.

Beasley, D. S., and Shriner, T. H.: Auditory analysis of temporally distorted sentential approximations. *Audio, 12*(4): 262-271, 1973.

Berlin, C. I., Lowe-Bell, S. S., Cullen, J. K., Jr., Thompson, C. L., and Loovis, C. F.: Dichotic speech perception an interpretation or right-ear advantage and temporal offset effects. *J Acoust Soc Am, 53*(3): 699-709, 1973.

Bernstein, B.: *Everyday Problems and the Child with Learning Difficulties.* New York, John Day, 1967.

Boder, E.: Developmental dyslexia: A diagnostic approach based on three atypical reading — spelling patterns. *Devel Med Child Neurol, 15*(5):663-685, 1973.

Bower, G. H. (Ed.): *Psychology of Learning and Motivation.* New York, Acad Pr, vol. 5, 1972.

Bradley, D. P.: Indentification and evaluation of the language characteristics of children with learning disabilities and implications for early intervention. *Div Child Commun Disord, 9*(1): 5-11, 1972.

Buchanan, A. R.: *Functional Neuro-Anatomy,* Philadelphia, Lea & Febiger, 1961.

Carrol, J. B.: *Language and Thought.* Englewood Cliffs, Foundations of Modern Psychology Series, P-H, 1964.

Chalfant, J. C., and Scheffelin, M. A.: *Central Processing Dysfunctions in Children:* A Review of Research, NINDS, Monograph No. 9, U.S. Dept. of H.E.W., 1969.

Douglas, R. J., and Pribram, K. H.: Learning and limbic lesions. *Neuropsychologia, 4:* 197-230, 1966.

Eisenberg, R. A.: The development of hearing in man: An assessment of current status. *ASHA, 12*(3): 119-123, 1970.

Feldman, R. B., Pinsky, L., Mendelson, J., and Lajoie, R.: Can language disorder not due to peripheral deafness be an isolated expression of prenatal rubella? *Pediatrics, 52*(2): 296-299, 1973.

Gardner, E.: *Fundamentals of Neurology.* Philadelphia, Saunders, 1968.
Getman, G. N.: *How To Develop Your Child's Intelligence.* Luverne, Announcer Pr, 1962.
Goldberg, H. K., and Schiffman, G. B.: *Dyslexia: Problems of Reading Disabilities.* New York, Grune, 1972.
Goodglass, H.: Developmental comparison of vowels and consonants in dichotic listening. *J Speech Hearing Res, 16*(4): 744-752, 1973.
Hagger, D.: Specific learning difficulties and deaf children. *Austral Teacher Deaf, 13*(1): 13-19, 1972.
John, E. R.: *Mechanisms of Memory.* New York, Acad Pr, 1967.
Johnson, D. J., and Myklebust, H. R.: *Learning Disabilities: Educational Principles and Practices.* New York, Grune, 1967.
Kavanagh, J. F., and Mattingly, I. G. (Eds.): *Language By Ear and By Eye.* Cambridge, MIT Pr, 1972.
Klasen, E.: *The Syndrome of Specific Dyslexia.* Baltimore, Univ Park Pr, 1972.
Kleffner, F. R.: *Language Disorders In Children,* Indianapolis, Bobbs, 1973.
Lafon, J. C.: Le developpement du langage: Language et naissances a haut risque. *J Franc ORL, 22*(5): 399-404, 1973.
Lawrence, J.: *Alpha Brain Waves,* New York, Avon, 1972.
Leventhal, G.: Effect of sentence context on word perception. *J Exp Psychol, 101*(2): 318-323, 1973.
Mandell, A. J., and Mandell, M. P.(Eds.): *Psychochemical Research In Man: Methods, Strategy and Theory.* New York, Acad Pr, 1969.
Mann, P. H., and Suiter, P.: *Handbook In Diagnostic Teaching: A Learning Disabilities Approach.* Boston, Allyn, 1974.
Mullin, T. A.: The effects of compressed and expanded speech on intelligibility in individuals with cerebrovascular accidents. Ph.D. dissertation, Syracuse University, 1971.
Murphy, J. F.: *Listening, Language, and Learning Disabilities.* Cambridge, Educators Publishing Service, Inc., 1970.
Mussen, P. H., Conger, J. J., and Kagan, J.: *Child Development and Personality.* New York, HarRow, 1969.
Myers, P. I., and Hammill, D. D.: *Methods For Learning Disorders.* New York, Wiley, 1969.
Myklebust, H. R. (Ed.): *Progress In Learning Disabilities.* New York, Grune, 1968, vol. 1, vol. 2, 1971.
Myklebust, H. R., and Boshes, B.: *Minimal Brain Damage in Children, Final Report.* Evanston, Northwestern Univ., 1969 (U. S. Public Health Service Contract 108-65-142.)
Norman, D. A. (Ed.): *Models of Human Memory,* New York, Acad Pr, 1970.
Pribram, K. H.: The limbic systems: Efferent control of neural inhibition and behavior. *Prog Brain Res, 27*: 318-336, 1967.
Russell, D. H.: *Children's Thinking.* Boston, Ginn & Co., 1956.
Rutherford, W. L.: From diagnosis to treatment of reading disabilities. *Acad Ther Q 8*(1): 51-55, 1972.

Shields, D. T.: Brain responses to stimuli in disorders of information processing. *J Learn Disabil, 6*(8): 501-505, 1973.

Sperry, V. B.: *A Language Approach To Learning Disabilities: A Source Book of Activities For Teachers.* Palo Alto, Cal., Consulting Psychologists Pr, 1972.

Taylor, I. G.: *Neurological Mechanisms of Hearing and Speech in Children,* Manchester, The University of Manchester Press, 1964.

Van Atta, B.: A comparative study of auditory skills (sensitivity, discrimination, and memroy span) of dyslalic and normal speaking children in grades 1-3. *AVISCO, 4*(1): 1-7, 1973.

Weston, A. J. (Ed.): *Communicative Disorders: An appraisal.* Springfield, Thomas, 1972.

Wiig, E. H. and Semel, E. M.: Comprehension of linguistic concepts requiring logical operations by learning disabled children. *J Speech Hearing Res, 16*(4): 627-636, 1973.

Wilson, J. A. R., Robeck, M. D., and Michael, W. B.: *Psychological Foundations of Learning and Teaching.* New York, McGraw, 1969.

Wunderlich, R. C.: *Allergy, Brains, and Children Coping.* St. Petersburg, Johnny Reads, 1973.

Zaner, A. R., Levee, R. F., and Guinta, R. R.: The development of auditory perceptual skills as a function of maturation: A pilot study. *J Aud Res, 8*: 313-322, 1968.

GLOSSARY

ACTH — Adrenocorticotrophic hormone, a pituitary gland hormone that stimulates the cortex of the adrenal glands.

Air conduction — The process by which sound is conducted to the inner ear (cochlea) via the air medium.

Ambient noise level — The audible alterations in air pressure caused by the everpresent noise of the environment.

Amplitude — Air pressure increase at a given point during the occurrence of sound.

Amygdala — A portion of the limbic system consisting of a mass of gray matter in the anterior portion of the temporal lobe. It appears to play an important function in conditioning and learning and to have a mutually inhibitory relationship with the reticular formation in the process of arousal and attention, thus determining what memories are to be laid down (along with the hippocampus).

Anoxia — Oxygen deficiency.

Auditory evoked potential — An acoustically-stimulated electrical change, recorded from a specific part of the brain (electroencephalic audiometry or EEA).

Auditory feedback — Return of one's speech auditorily (both via air and bone conduction). To hear oneself talking. Because the distance between the ear and mouth is fairly constant, varying little with growth and age, one hears one's own speech as being more highly resonant (sonorous) than it actually is.

Auditory figure-ground discrimination — The ability to shift attention between two sources of auditory stimuli, the primary stimulus becoming the figure with the secondary stimulus becoming the ground.

Auditory pathways — Major synaptic junctions of the VIII cranial nerve located in the medulla and pons areas of the brain stem (in ascending order):
1. Ventral and dorsal cochlear nuclei (medulla)
2. Superior olivary complex (medulla)
3. Inferior colliculi (pons)
4. Medial geniculate bodies (hindbrain)

Autonomic Nervous System (ANS) — Division of nervous system which serves to regulate smooth muscle and glandular activity. The activities of the ANS are primarily free from voluntary control. They can be consciously influenced, however, from the brain and through the spinal cord. The two divisions of the ANS are the sympathetic and parasympathetic.

Bone conduction — The process by which sound is conducted to the nerve of hearing through the cranial bones.

Brain stem — Areas of the axial portion of the brain exclusive of the cerebrum and cerebellum; this portion includes the pons and medulla oblongata.

Cerebral cortex (gray matter) — Outer superficial gray mantel of the cerebral hemispheres. Contains about 14 billion cells and about 200 million incoming and outgoing projection fibers and six layers of laminae or cells.

Corticosteroids — Steroid substances obtained from the cortex of the adrenal gland.

Decibel (dB) — A useful measurement for comparing the loudness of two sounds. The decibel is logarithm of a ratio of two values of power, and equal changes in dB represent equal ratios.

End organ — The end organ of hearing is the organ of Corti within the cochlea where sound stimuli are transduced into electrochemical impulses to be interpreted and acted upon by the brain.

Engram — A memory trace caused by a protoplasmic change in neural tissue within the brain and brain stem hypothesized to account for the persistence of memory.

Folic acid — Pteroylglutamic acid. Found in liver, yeast and green leaves.

Free field — In practice, a region exercising little negative effect over the sound stimuli induced (see sound field).

Frequency (Hz, Hertz) — The number of complete cycles occurring in a second of time. Any variation in the frequency of a sound is usually accompanied by a variation in the pitch of the sound.

Frontal lobe — Main area of cortex responsible for motor activities, personality and intellect (anterior areas). Located in front of the fissure of Rolando (central sulcus).

High-pass filter — A wave filter with a single transmission band, extending from a cutoff frequency up to approximately 10,000 Hz.

Hippocampus — Most medial portion of the cerebral cortex. This portion of the limbic system is important in laying down permanent memory traces by storing recent memory patterns and segments of behavioral patterns where they are both free from disruption by distracting influences and where they are nevertheless immediately available to those mechanisms actually organizing ongoing behavior or permanent memory formation.

Hypothalamus — Situated beneath the thalamus, it contains neurosecretions which are important in the control of visceral activities such as maintenance of water balance, sugar and fat metabolism, regulation of body temperature and secretion of endocrine glands.

Infantile autism — Severe disassociation or withdrawal from interpersonal relationships.

Low-pass filter — A wave filter with a single transmission band extending from zero frequency up to some cutoff frequency.

Minimal brain dysfunction — " . . . refers to children of near average, average or above average general intelligence, with certain learning or behavioral disabilities ranging from mild to severe, which are associated with deviations of function of the CNS. These deviations may manifest themselves by various combinations of impairment in perception, conceptualization, language, memory, and control of attention, impulse or motor function." (Clements, 1966).

Narrow-band masking noise — A masking noise having most of its energy within a narrow, definable band, usually at one-half octave above and one-half octave below a given frequency.

Neocortex — The nonolfactory portion of the cerebral cortex.

Neurohumoral imbalance — An imbalance (increase or decrease) in the amount of chemical transmitter in the nervous system.

Norepinephrine — A biogenic amine at the synapses in the brain believed to be a key neurotransmitter or modulator in the CNS.

Occipital lobe — Cortical area primarily responsible for visual functions. Located posterior to the occipitoparietal fissure.

Parietal Lobe — Main cortical area for the discrimination of size, shape, body position in space, body movement awareness, and so on. Located above the fissure of Sylvius (lateral cerebral fissure) and behind the fissure of Rolando.

Phonetically balanced word list (PB) — Lists of fifty monosyllabic words scientifically chosen so that each list contains samples of speech sounds in the same proportion with which they occur in English speech.

Prenatal — occurring or existing before birth.

Psycholinguistic approach — The approach which combines the fields of behavioral psychology and linguistics. The approach is based on the principles that (1) behavioral psychology can provide teaching methods which will facilitate language learning and (2) a sound linguistic basis can provide the systematic analysis and description to guide the content and order or presentation of the linguistic elements to be taught.

Psychotropic drugs — Substances capable of influencing psychological and mental processes and of modifying emotions and behavior.

Reticular formation — Reticular nuclei associated with bidirectional tracts connecting all levels of the brain stem with the cerebral cortex. The entire system constitutes the activating and integrating system which promotes motivation, attention and facilitation-inhibition in coding. The formation extends from the medulla oblongata to the thalamus in the midbrain.

Reverberation time — The time in seconds for the sound level in a room to drop 60 dB (or a drop to one-millionth of its previous intensity).

Rhinencephalic-midbrain complex — Includes olfactory bulb, olfactory tract and striae, intermediate olfactory area, pyriform area, paraterminal area, hippocampal formation and fornix. It constitutes the paleopallium and archipallium.

Schizophrenia — A cleavage of fissure of the mental functions (dementia praecox).

Sound field — A defined region containing sound waves transmitted through loudspeakers rather than earphones.

Stimulus plexus — Coincidental stimuli which are susceptible to discrimination as to their relative importance or value.

Strabismus — Inability to direct both eyes to the same object, due to incoordination of the eye muscles.

Syndrome — A set of symptoms occurring together, especially associated with central nervous system disorders.

Temporal lobe — Area of cortex primarily responsible for auditory functions. Located below the fissure of Sylvius and continuous posteriorly with the occipital lobe.

Thalamus — The largest subdivision of the diencephalon. All sensory impulses, with the exception of olfactory impulses, are received by the thalamus. These are associated and synthesized, then relayed through the thalamocortical radiations to the specific cortical areas.

Toxemia — Absorption of bacterial products or toxins formed at a source of infection.

Transnatal (Perinatal) — Occurring shortly before or after birth.

White noise — A noise whose spectrum level is substantially independent of frequency over a specified range.

INDEX